Removable Orthodontic Appliances

K. G. Isaacson F.D.S., M.Orth R.C.S. Eng.
Consultant Orthodontist, North Hampshire Hospital, Basingstoke, UK

J. D. Muir B.D.S., F.D.S., M.Orth R.C.S. Eng.
Consultant Orthodontist, North Staffordshire Hospital, Stoke-on-Trent, UK

and

R. T. Reed B.D.S., F.D.S.R.C.P.S. Glas. M.Orth R.C.S. Eng.
Consultant Orthodontist, North Hampshire Hospital, Basingstoke, UK

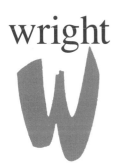

wright

OXFORD AUCKLAND BOSTON JOHANNESBURG MELBOURNE NEW DELHI

Wright
An imprint of Elsevier Science

First published 2002

British Library Cataloguing in Publication Data
A catalogue reference for this book is available from the British Library

Library of Congress Cataloguing in Publication Data
A catalogue reference for this book is available from the Library of Congress

ISBN 0 7236 1053 3

For information on all Wright's publications visit
our website at www.bh.com/dentistry-wright

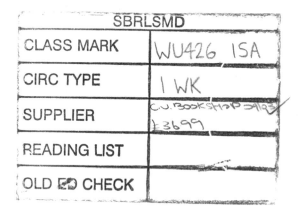
Composition by Scribe Design, Gillingham, Kent
Printed and bound in Great Britain by MPG Books Ltd, Bodmin, Cornwall

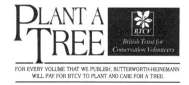

FOR EVERY VOLUME THAT WE PUBLISH, BUTTERWORTH-HEINEMANN
WILL PAY FOR BTCV TO PLANT AND CARE FOR A TREE.

Contents

Contents of CD ROM

Acknowledgements

The authors and publishers would like to acknowledge gratefully the support and help they have received from Orthocare in the production of the accompanying CD ROM. Thanks are also due to Professor J. Sandy, Bristol University; Mr G. Lucas, Information technology advisor, Wessex Postgraduate Dental Deanery; and Mr G. Ashton, Senior chief orthodontic technician, North Hampshire Hospital, Basingstoke.

Illustrations

The Authors are responsible for the illustrations. They are intended to be diagrammatic and wire dimensions are not necessarily to scale.

Preface

At the start of a new century, publication of a book on removable appliances may be unexpected. But, despite a great increase in the use of fixed appliances the majority of courses of orthodontic treatment in the United Kingdom are still carried out with removable appliances. In General and Specialist practice within the National Health Service the number of courses of treatment carried out with removable appliances is in the order of 400,000 appliances each year. A recent survey showed that even the Hospital Service of the United Kingdom (which concentrates on the management of more severe malocclusions) uses removable appliances in 16% of cases – frequently in combination with fixed and functional appliances.

We make no suggestion that removable appliances are suitable for the treatment of every patient. But their careful use, in selected cases, can contribute to effective treatment which produces acceptable results.

We hope that this book will improve the results that can be achieved and make practitioners more aware of those patients who require more complex techniques and referral to a specialist.

This book is a combination of two previous books: *Orthodontic Treatment with Removable Appliances* by Houston and Isaacson and *Tooth Movement with Removable Appliances* by Muir and Reed. Both of these sold widely in the United Kingdom and overseas and were translated into a number of languages. When reprints were considered it was thought that a joint work would combine the strengths of both previous books. This book includes a CD ROM showing the clinical records of patients treated with the use of removable appliances.

It was a privilege for us to know, and work with, the late Professor Bill Houston, whom we regard as one of the United Kingdom's leading orthodontic teachers and research-workers during the twentieth century.

K.G. Isaacson
J.D. Muir
R.T. Reed

Chapter 1

Introduction

Removable appliances are, by definition, orthodontic appliances that can be inserted and removed by the patient. They comprise a number of components, each of which will be described, along with their clinical uses, in separate chapters.

Removable appliances began to be used routinely in the 19th century, but these were relatively crude devices, constructed from vulcanite, with precious metal wires and sometimes depending for their action on the expansion of hickory wood pegs when soaked by saliva. Complex removable appliances, often relying upon the action of expansion screws, were evolved in the early part of the 20th century.

Modern removable appliances generally use acrylic baseplates and stainless steel wires. With the development by Adams of the modified arrowhead clasp (1950) the scope and efficiency of these appliances was greatly increased. Unfortunately, they often represented the only available method of treatment and, as a result, were commonly used to treat a wide range of malocclusions for which they were inadequate and unsuited. In recent years fixed appliance techniques have been transformed, particularly with the introduction of pre-formed bands and components, direct bonding techniques, pre-adjusted brackets and, more recently, by the advent of pre-formed archwires in stainless steel as well as non-ferrous alloys. These advances, coupled with the growth of orthodontic specialization, have inevitably diminished the role of the removable appliance, but it may, nevertheless, continue to be the appliance of choice for selected cases. Removable appliances can also have a role in combination with fixed appliances and can be particularly useful in carrying out local, interceptive tooth movements in the mixed dentition. They are effective space maintainers and are used almost universally as retention appliances after the completion of active tooth movements for cases treated with fixed appliances.

In some areas of clinical activity, removable appliances have significant advantages over fixed appliances. A well-constructed maxillary removable appliance can be highly conservative of anchorage. Intraoral anchorage is not only provided by the teeth themselves but also supplemented by the contact of the acrylic baseplate with the palatal vault. This is particularly useful where it is necessary to achieve occlusal movement of misplaced or impacted teeth, for example in the correction of unerupted incisors and canines. Traction can be applied to these teeth to bring them down to the occlusal level using the palate as anchorage. A fixed appliance is, by contrast, much more likely to intrude and tip the adjacent teeth. Inexperienced practitioners often assume that removable appliances demand little skill and that their design can safely be left to the laboratory. In reality, considerable skill is required. If an appliance is to be exploited to its full potential it must be thoughtfully designed, well constructed and carefully supervised. The general practitioner can, with suitable training, use removable appliances successfully to deal with simpler cases, but the specialist will still find their use invaluable.

Action of removable appliances

Functional appliances are sometimes considered as 'removable appliances'. (They are, of course, almost always removable) but they depend for their effect on maintaining the mandible in a postured position, influencing both the orofacial musculature and dentoalveolar development. They are beyond the scope of this volume, which will deal only with simple removable appliances.

Spontaneous movement

Where extractions are carried out as part of treatment, the relief of crowding may, on its own, allow neighbouring teeth to upright towards the extraction sites. Removable appliances can enhance such tooth movement and treatment depends principally upon the ability of the active components of the appliance to tip teeth. In many cases, spontaneous tooth movement can be relied upon to assist alignment and this may be particularly important in the lower arch, where removable appliances are bulky and are less efficient.

Because spontaneous tooth movement is so important as an adjunct to removable appliance treatment, significant factors relating to spontaneous tooth movement are considered below.

Eruption guidance

In the late mixed dentition stage, appropriate extractions allow an enhanced path of eruption for crowded or misplaced teeth. Removable appliances have an important role to play as space maintainers, following relief of crowding. This is considered fully in Chapter 7 on class I malocclusions.

Uprighting

When crowding is relieved a tooth may upright by movement of the crown towards an adjacent extraction space (Figure 1.1). This is commonly associated with crowding of canines and works most effectively when the crowns are mesially

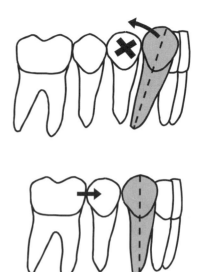

Figure 1.1 Spontaneous uprighting of a mesially inclined lower canine following extraction of a lower first premolar.

inclined because uprighting can take place towards the first premolar extraction sites. In the lower arch this can be particularly beneficial.

Labio-lingual movement

(a) Anterior teeth

The lower labial segment may be influenced by soft tissue contact from the tongue and lips. The tongue provides an anterior component of force to lingually displaced incisors while the lips provide a lingually directed force to proclined or labially crowded incisors (Figure 1.2). These forces may permit considerable spontaneous alignment of imbricated lower incisors once crowding has been relieved. The effect is much less marked in the upper arch because the tongue does not contact the upper incisors to the same extent.

(b) Posterior teeth

There is limited soft tissue influence in the bucco-lingual position of the upper posterior teeth but, in the lower posterior segments, impacted second premolars are often uprighted by the action of the tongue once crowding has been relieved, provided there is no cuspal interlocking. Upper removable appliances often

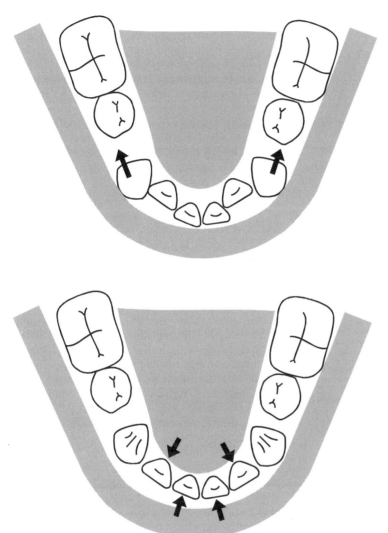

Figure 1.2 Alignment of a crowded lower labial segment can occur spontaneously in a growing patient following the relief of crowding.

assist spontaneous alignment in the lower arch by virtue of the fact that biteplates can be used to unlock the occlusion.

Mesial migration

Natural mesial drift of the posterior teeth occurs at any age but is more marked in the growing child. If extraction treatment is being considered this may represent an advantage or a disadvantage. It is a disadvantage when space is barely adequate. It is an advantage whenever the extractions will create excessive space and particularly so in the lower arch, where mesial movement can not only assist in the closure of first premolar spaces but may also allow the

lower molars to move forwards from a class II towards a class I relationship (Figure 1.3). This change can sometimes be maximized by carrying out lower extractions in advance of upper extractions to establish a class 1 molar relationship early in treatment.

At the end of removable appliance treatment residual extraction space will often remain. This is a common target for criticism of the standard of removable appliance results but, provided that spaces are matching, not excessive and that the cuspal relationships are correct, the spacing will usually improve subsequently in a growing patient.

In the upper arch spontaneous mesial movement of buccal teeth can also assist space

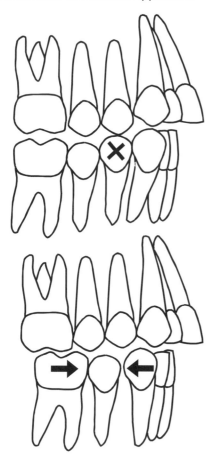

Figure 1.3 Relief of crowding in the lower arch in advance of the upper arch can allow for the establishment of a class I molar relationship.

closure. Unfortunately, the readiness with which such movement occurs can exacerbate any anchorage loss produced by injudicious appliance use.

Timing of spontaneous movement

Spontaneous movement takes place while the patient is growing and may occur most rapidly during the pubertal growth spurt, when there is a considerable amount of bone development and remodelling. From a practical point of view, the majority of labio-lingual and uprighting movements will take place within a 6-month period following extractions. Where space is obviously excessive it may be wise to allow some initial closure before fitting the first

appliance. After that time, appliance treatment may be considered if there has been insufficient spontaneous change. Frequently, a removable appliance may be used in the upper arch when the lower arch either requires no treatment or will align spontaneously following premolar extractions.

If the capacity for spontaneous tooth movement is fully utilized throughout treatment then the range of cases which can be treated with removable appliances will be extended and the standard of results improved.

Active movements

Tipping

Removable appliances act by applying controlled forces to the crowns of the teeth. Because only single-point contact is possible, tooth movement occurs solely by tipping (Figure 1.4). The fulcrum will usually be about 40% down the length of the root from the apex. By applying forces of 25–50 g, tipping can be achieved with the crown moving by about 1 mm per month. Active removable appliances should be used only where the teeth can be tipped into their correct positions.

Tipping can either be in a mesio-distal direction (in the line of the arch) or in a bucco-palatal direction. The key feature is the position of the apex of the tooth before movement. When the apex is well positioned, a tooth will usually respond satisfactorily to removable appliance treatment provided that the direction of movement tends to upright it. A tooth which

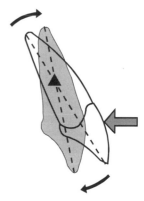

Figure 1.4 Application of a force to the crown of the tooth results in a tipping movement.

is tipped unfavourably, for instance a distally inclined canine, will not respond satisfactorily to further distal movement with a removable appliance.

Mesio-distal tipping

Teeth can be tipped towards a space, usually one which has been created by extraction to relieve crowding. Where a tooth is mesially inclined it can be readily tipped and uprighted. The commonest example of such tooth movement is provided by the retraction of canines. Upright or distally inclined canines will become more distally inclined as the result of tipping with a removable appliance. A decision has to be made as to how much retraction will be acceptable. There is some evidence that teeth which have been tipped with a removable appliance will undergo limited uprighting in the post-treatment period (Brenchley, 1966).

Bucco-lingual tipping

Bucco-lingual movement of incisors can be carried out readily, but in the lower arch, the labio-lingual position of the incisors is normally accepted. Movement should only be sufficient to compensate for crowding of the lower incisors and deliberate proclination of the lower labial segment is highly likely to relapse.

In the upper arch, tipping of the upper incisors can readily be accomplished with a removable appliance. The essential criterion must be the position of the apices of the incisors, which will only alter slightly when tipping takes place. Retraction of the incisors in a mild class II occlusion or labial movement of the crowns in a mild class III occlusion can be readily achieved (Figure 1.5). Buccal movement of the upper posterior teeth is much more difficult to accomplish, except in crossbite cases associated with a displacement activity of the mandible.

Rotations and controlled apical movements

Such movements require two-point contact on the crown of the tooth. Many attempts have been made to design removable appliances that will achieve this, but they are not generally

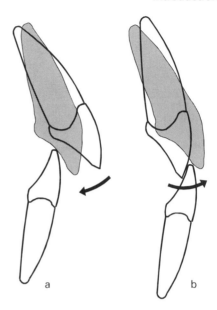

Figure 1.5 Tipping of the upper incisors. (a) In a palatal direction, can correct a mild class II case. (b) In a labial direction, can correct a mild class III case.

successful. This is because it is difficult to maintain a controlled, well-positioned force-couple on a tooth as it moves. Unwanted effects, such as tilting and elongation, are also prone to occur. Where a bonded fixed attachment is used it is possible to correct the rotation of a single tooth with a removable appliance. Commonly, however, a rotation may be combined with an apical malposition and unless this can also be controlled the result may still be unsatisfactory.

Occlusal movement

To achieve such movement it is necessary to provide a point of attachment for an occlusally directed force on the crown of the tooth. An attachment bonded to the crown makes it relatively simple to do this with a removable appliance, particularly at the front of the arch (Figure 1.6).

Intrusion

Relative intrusion of groups of teeth (particularly of the lower labial segment) can be achieved by contact with an appliance fitted in the opposing arch. This is frequently invaluable because it means that an increased, complete

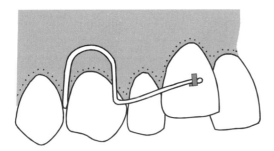

Figure 1.6 A bonded attachment on the labial surface of an upper incisor allows occlusal movement with a buccally placed spring.

producing a 'functional' effect. (Fixed appliance systems would demand a separate, lower appliance to achieve such changes.) For such an improvement to be effective, it is desirable that facial growth should be taking place.

In a class II division I malocclusion, proclined upper incisors frequently conceal an element of over-eruption which will demand intrusion as well as retraction. This is an indication for a fixed appliance and any attempts to use a removable appliance merely to tilt the upper incisors palatally risks producing an unsatisfactory and 'toothy' appearance.

overbite may be corrected during canine retraction, so allowing the upper incisors to be retracted on a subsequent appliance (Figure 1.7). In this respect the anterior bite plane is

Lower arch treatment

Removable appliances have limited use in the lower arch for a number of reasons:

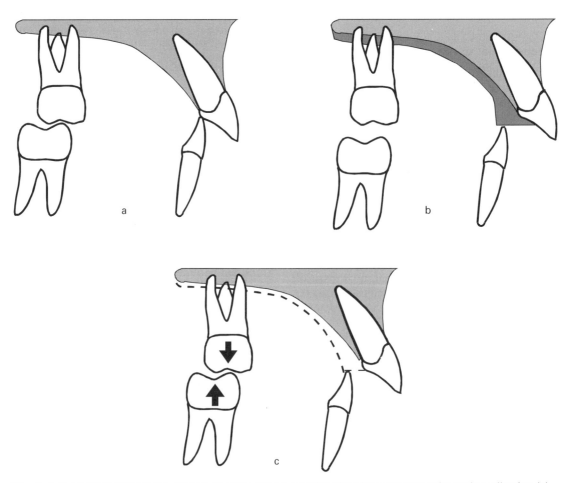

Figure 1.7 (a) An increased overjet and overbite. (b) An anterior bite plane separates the molars allowing (c) vertical eruption of the molar teeth, effectively reducing the overbite.

- Patients find that the bulk is unsatisfactory
- With conventional clasping techniques the retention is less satisfactory and this contributes to a patient's dislike of the appliance
- The considerably reduced area available for active components means that it is not possible to construct springs with a sufficiently long range of action.

Case selection

Age of patient

Removable appliances are most suitable for use between the ages of 6 and 16 years, with the majority of treatment undertaken during the late mixed and early permanent dentition stages.

Dental factors

In some malocclusions, the positions of the tooth apices are relatively correct and the irregularity is due to the crowns being tipped from the correct positions. Such cases are most suited to treatment by removable appliances because tipping movements are required. For the relief of moderate crowding, extractions should be close to the site where space is needed. Cases that require controlled space closure, for example where mild crowding is to be treated by second premolar extractions, are not suitable for the use of removable appliances. Severe crowding, multiple rotations or marked apical displacement of teeth are also inappropriate for removable appliance treatment. Spacing, except where it is associated with an increased overjet, cannot usually be dealt with by removable appliances alone.

Crossbites, especially those associated with a displacement, may be effectively treated with removable appliances where the use of occlusal coverage eliminates the displacement. Excessive overbites or marked anterior open bites are not suitable for management with removable appliances alone.

Skeletal factors

Cases with class I, mild or moderate class II and very mild class III skeletal patterns are suitable for management. Removable appliances are not suitable for the complete treatment of more marked class II or class III cases.

Summary

Removable appliances can be used to treat a large number of mild and moderate malocclusions, especially in the growing patient where the lower arch is acceptable or will improve spontaneously following relief of crowding. They are also useful for the reduction of overbite, the elimination of displacements and the provision of additional anchorage. They can provide a ready adjunct to other forms of treatment, especially treatment with fixed appliances where they are almost routinely used as removable retainers when active tooth movement is completed.

References

Brenchley, M.L. (1966) Some spontaneous and advantageous tooth movements. *Dental Practitioner*, **16**: 307–311

Further reading

Adams, C.P., Kerr, W.J.S. (1990) *Design construction and use of removable appliances.* Wright, London
British Orthodontic Society (1998) *Young practitioners guide to orthodontics.* British Orthodontic Society, London
Isaacson, K.G., Reed, R.T., Stephens, C.D. (1990) *Functional orthodontic appliances.* Blackwell, Oxford
Littlewood, S.J., Tait, A.G., Mandall, N.A., Lewis, D.H. (2001) The role of removable appliances in contemporary orthodontics. *British Dental Journal*, **191**: 304–310
Proffitt, W.R. (2000) *Contemporay orthodontics*, 3rd edn. Mosby, St Louis
Russell, J.I. *et al.* (1999) The consultant orthodontic service. *British Dental Journal*, **187**: 149–153
Stephens, C.D., Isaacson, K.G. (1990) *Practical orthodontic assessment.* Heinemann, Oxford
Turbill, E.A., Richmond, S., Wright, J.L. (1999) A closer look at general dental service orthodontics in England & Wales. *British Dental Journal*, **187**: 271–274
Williams, J.K., Cook, P.A., Isaacson, K.G., Thom, A.R. (1995) *Fixed orthodontic appliances – principles and practice.* Wright, Oxford.

Chapter 2

Biomechanics of tooth movement

When a force is applied to the crown of a tooth, it will be displaced slightly within the confines of the periodontal ligament. Depending on the type of force applied, the tooth may be tipped, moved bodily, or rotated about its long axis (Figure 2.1). This small change in tooth position will set up areas of tension and compression within the periodontal ligament. Provided that the force is applied over a sufficient period of time, remodelling of the socket wall will allow the tooth to move further.

An understanding of these processes is of clinical relevance in that the rationale of appliance adjustment is based on our knowledge of them.

Tooth movements

When a force is applied to a point on a smooth surface, it can be resolved into two components, one at right angles to the surface and the

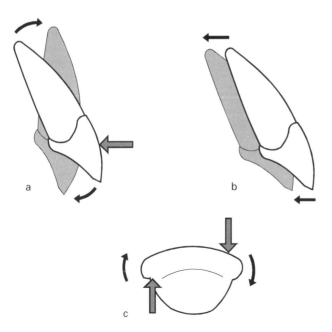

Figure 2.1 Three kinds of tooth movement. (a) Tipping. (b) Bodily movement. (c) Rotation about the long axis.

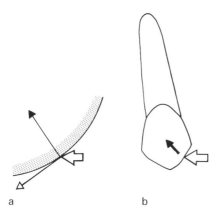

a   b

Figure 2.2 (a) When a force is applied to a curved surface, the direction of the resultant movement is at right angles to the tangent at the point of contact. (b) A partially erupted tooth will be intruded if a spring is applied to the cuspal incline.

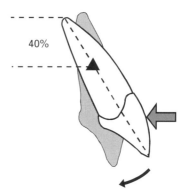

Figure 2.3 When a tooth is tipped with a removable appliance, the fulcrum of rotation is approximately 40% of the length of the root from the apex.

other parallel to it (Figure 2.2). Where the surface is curved, the force is resolved perpendicular and parallel to the tangent at the point of contact. If the force is applied at an angle to the surface, tooth movement will be produced by the perpendicular component. Thus, the tooth will not move in the direction of the applied force.

Although the initial movement must be considered in three dimensions, it is convenient to discuss it in the two planes which span the space: first the plane through the long axis of the tooth and in the direction of tooth movement, and second, a plane of cross-section.

Movements in the plane of the long axis

When a force is applied to the crown of a tooth, movement is resisted by the periodontal ligament.

Tipping movements

A force applied at a single point on the crown will tip the tooth about a fulcrum. Although many texts suggest that tipping takes place about a fulcrum within the apical third of the root, it can be shown that the centre of rotation is usually about 40% of the length of the root from the apex (Christiansen and Burstone, 1969). This means that while the crown moves

in one direction, the apex moves in the opposite direction (Figure 2.3). The exact level of the fulcrum depends on a number of factors, which are not under control of the orthodontist: these include root shape and the distribution of fibre bundles within the periodontal ligament.

Bodily movements

If a tooth is to be moved bodily, a force couple must be applied to the crown in conjunction with the original force (Figure 2.4). This would be necessary to allow precise control over the position of the fulcrum but is not normally a practical undertaking with removable appliances. It is possible with fixed appliances and, to a very limited extent, with fixed components used in conjunction with removable appliances.

Intrusion

When a bite plane is incorporated in an appliance, an intrusive force is applied to the teeth which contact it. The amount of true intrusion is small and overbite reduction with removable appliances is largely the result of eruption of the posterior teeth (Figure 2.5). Where an incisor does not occlude perpendicular to an anterior bite plane, it may be tipped labially.

Intrusion of teeth may also be produced unintentionally by the incorrect application of a spring. Where, for example, a spring to retract a canine is applied to the cuspal incline, the tooth will be intruded as well as retracted. This most often happens when attempts are made to retract a canine which has only partially

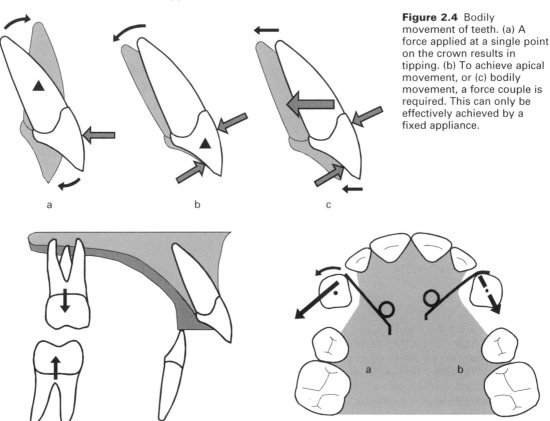

Figure 2.4 Bodily movement of teeth. (a) A force applied at a single point on the crown results in tipping. (b) To achieve apical movement, or (c) bodily movement, a force couple is required. This can only be effectively achieved by a fixed appliance.

a   b   c

Figure 2.5 An anterior bite plane allows vertical development of the posterior teeth.

Figure 2.6 Application of force to the crown of a tooth. (a) The palatal cantilever spring is positioned too far posteriorly, the tooth will be moved buccally. The point of contact of the spring is also incorrect resulting in unwanted rotation of the canine. (b) Correct application of a palatal finger spring to a canine.

erupted. For this reason, it is preferable not to attempt to move a tooth until it has erupted fully.

Movements in the plane of the occlusion

The example selected in this discussion is the retraction of an upper canine, but the argument applies equally to other situations.

The tooth will move in the direction of the component of force perpendicular to its surface. This is of particular importance when considering tooth movement in this plane. It is common to find that the spring is positioned too far posteriorly, so that the resultant force does not lie in the required direction along the line of the arch, but is directed buccally (Figure 2.6). The tooth will then move buccally as well

as distally. The unwanted buccal movement is particularly difficult to avoid when the tooth is buccally positioned in the first place. In these circumstances, a buccal spring, which can apply a force at the required point, is essential.

If the resultant force does not pass through the long axis of the tooth, a rotation will be induced. Rotations of this sort may be particularly difficult to avoid if the tooth is already slightly rotated. Teeth in this position must be controlled by a spring which can apply the force from a buccal direction.

Rotations

While rotations may inadvertently be introduced as described above, the controlled rotation of a tooth can only be undertaken with a couple. With an upper central incisor, it may be possible to correct a rotation with a couple between a labial bow and a palatal spring at the baseplate, but this requires careful management.

Tissue changes during tooth movement

As a result of the initial tooth movement described above, areas of compression and tension are set up within the periodontal ligament. The distribution of these areas depends on the nature of the initial tooth movement. If the tooth tips, the pressure varies along the root, being greatest at the alveolar crest and apex. It should be remembered that the pressure at any level will vary with the width of the periodontal ligament and around the circumference of the root. With bodily tooth movement, which is not possible with simple removable appliances, the distribution of pressure is more uniform along the root length, but still varies around the circumference. The more uniform distribution of pressure with bodily tooth movements means that for a given force applied to the crown of a tooth, the maximal pressure (and tension), within the periodontal ligament will be less than with tipping movements.

In response to these changes in pressure induced in the periodontal ligament, tissue changes take place. The nature of the changes depends on whether the area in question is one of compression or tension and whether capillary blood pressure is exceeded locally.

Areas of compression

Where capillary blood pressure is not exceeded

In this case there may be local changes in blood flow, but the capillaries remain patent. An increase in cellular proliferation takes place, both in the fibroblasts of the periodontal ligament and among the osteoprogenitor cells, which line the socket. The stimulus for proliferation of the osteoprogenitor cells, which eventually results in increased bone formation, is seen on the tension side. On the pressure side,

osteoclasts are recruited to cause bone resorption in the area of pressure. The stimulus for the recruitment and activation of osteoclasts is thought to arise from the mechanical perturbation of the osteoblast which then signals to the osteoclast to increase its activity. The vascularity is an important aspect of these changes since osteoclasts are thought to form by fusion of circulating monocytes. A patent and intact blood vessel is therefore needed adjacent to the site of resorption since this is where the bone resorbing cells are recruited. Within a few days active resorption progresses so that the osteoclasts come to lie in shallow depressions (Howship's lacunae) on the bone surface.

The integrity of the periodontal ligament is maintained by the turnover of periodontal fibres. Fibroblasts are responsible for the formation of collagen and the ligament comprises 80% type I collagen and a significant level (15–20%) of type III collagen. The breakdown of these collagens is through a family of enzymes called the matrix metalloproteinases (MMPs) and their activity is balanced by the natural inhibitors of MMPs, the so-called tissue inhibitors of metalloproteinases (TIMPS). Eventually, direct surface resorption gradually remodels the socket wall and allows the tooth to move.

The tissue changes are not confined to the periodontal ligament and socket wall: within the canellous spaces of the bone, remodelling changes occur and on the external alveolar surface periosteal appositon of bone maintains the thickness of the alveolar process (Figure 2.7).

Where capillary blood pressure is locally exceeded

The capillaries are occluded, cells in the periodontal ligament die and on a histological level, the area becomes structureless or 'hyalinized'. The hyaline material is merely compressed collagenous tissue. Bone resorption depends both on a blood supply and on a cellular response. Neither of these is present in hyalinized areas and so direct surface resorption of bone is not possible. The areas of hyalinization are often quite localized. Deep to these areas (within the cancellous spaces of the alveolar bone) and peripherally (in surrounding areas of the periodontal ligament which are compressed, but not hyalinized), osteoclastic

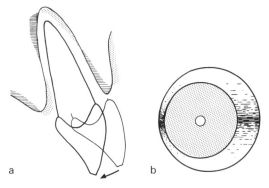

a   b

Figure 2.7 (a) Areas of bone resorption (stipple) and apposition (horizontal shading) associated with orthodontic tipping movement. (b) Pressure in the periodontal ligament varies around the circumference of the root.

action takes place. This gradually removes the bone associated with the hyalinized area. When this has been done, the tooth is free to move. If the force applied is still excessive, a further hyalinized area will be set up against the newly exposed bone surface: but if the pressure is now below capillary blood pressure, the hyalinized area will be invaded by blood vessels and cells and direct surface resorption will then take place.

Areas of tension

The width of the periodontal ligament is increased by the initial tooth movement. Within a short period of time there is a proliferation of the fibroblasts of the periodontal ligament and of the osteoprogenitor cells in the socket wall. In areas of tension, these osteoprogenitor cells differentiate to become osteoblasts which lay down bone matrix (osteoid tissue). This osteoid tissue rapidly becomes calcified to form loose, vascular, woven bone. Over a period of months, the woven bone is remodelled to form mature trabeculae. Within the cancellous spaces remodelling of bone takes place and on the external surface of the alveolar process, periosteal resorption of bone is found. Thus the alveolar process drifts in the direction in which the tooth is moving. The fibres of the periodontal ligament are lengthened or reformed. Unlike the areas of compression, the

magnitude of the tension has only minor effects on the pattern of tissue activity. However, where the tension is excessive, periodontal fibres may be torn and capillaries ruptured so that there is haemorrhage into the periodontal ligament.

Biochemical

The biochemical aspects of tooth movement are complex and are beyond the scope of this book. The reader is referred to papers by Hill (1998), Sandy *et al.* (1993) and McDonald (1993) for further details.

The supra-alveolar connective tissues

Unlike the principal fibres of the periodontal ligament which pass between tooth and bone, the trans-septal and free gingival fibres do not rapidly re-adapt to the new tooth position. This is well illustrated by the rotation of teeth. Reitan (1967) has shown that the principal fibres become realigned within a few months, but the free gingival and other supra-alveolar connective tissue fibres remain under tension for considerable periods of time (Figure 2.8). The residual tension in these fibre systems may contribute to relapse following orthodontic rotation.

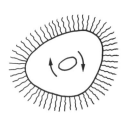

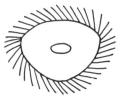

Figure 2.8 When a tooth is rotated about its long axis, the supra-alveolar connective tissues remain under tension.

Individual variation

There is considerable variation between individuals in bone density. In the majority of cases there are large cancellous spaces within the alveolar bone, whereas in a few individuals the bone is dense with very sparse cancellous spaces. Very dense bone of this type will be resorbed only slowly. This is of particular importance if areas of hyalinization are produced in the periodontal ligament. In cases with a dense bone, there will be little undermining resorption and if the area of hyalinization is extensive, it may be a considerable time before the bone is resorbed from the periphery. Individuals with this type of alveolar bone are quite rare, but if, on a radiograph, the bone structure appears to be very dense, active treatment with removable appliances should be minimized and very light forces should be used to move the teeth. A similar problem arises where a tooth, often an upper permanent canine, is buccally displaced and surrounded by a dense cortical plate. In these circumstances, priority should be given to moving the tooth into the line of the arch where it can be retracted more readily.

Age

Teeth can be moved orthodontically at any age. In the adult, the periodontal ligament is less cellular than in the growing child, and so the tissue changes may take longer to get under way. In addition, the alveolar bone may be rather more dense and tooth movement will be a little slower. However, in general, variations between individuals in the rate of tooth movement are greater than the changes with age. The types of treatment which are slower in the adult are those which depend to some extent upon facial growth. For example, overbite reduction is more difficult in the adult and spontaneous movement of teeth following relief of crowding is much more limited after facial growth and occlusal development are complete.

The forces used in producing tooth movement

The variations in the physical properties of the periodontal ligament and in the pressure distribution within it, makes it impossible to relate directly the force applied to the crown with magnitude of the local pressure changes. There is undoubtedly some threshold of force below which tooth movement will not occur, but at least in the case of a continuously applied force, this must be quite low. Where possible, the force applied to the tooth should be low enough to avoid areas of hyalinization in the periodontal ligament. Reitan (1967) has shown that with bodily movement, because the pressure is more uniformly distributed over the root surface, it is possible to avoid hyalinization: but with tipping, some hyalinization is usually produced at the alveolar crest where pressure is maximal. However, with light forces, this area is small and once it has been removed, in 2 or 3 weeks, direct surface resorption will occur. If larger forces are used, the area of hyalinization will be greater, resorption will take longer and tooth movement will be delayed. When tooth movement eventually does occur, the tooth will become slightly loose. If the applied force continues to be excessive, further hyalinization and delay will follow. Other problems, such as loss of anchorage will arise if heavy forces are used.

On empirical grounds, it has been established that for tipping movements of single-rooted teeth, with minimal hyalinization, the force should fall in the range between 25 g and 40 g (approximately 1–1.5 oz), the lower figure being appropriate for teeth with short roots, such as lateral incisors. However, for the first 2 or 3 weeks of tooth movement, even lighter forces (about half the above values) should be used. Where a number of teeth with a large root area are to be moved, for example in the retraction of upper buccal segments, greater forces may be appropriate.

The rate of tooth movement

The rate of tooth movement varies between patients but, in general, a rate of at least 1 mm a month is considered to be satisfactory. However, if tooth movement is less than this, it is probable that something is wrong with the adjustment of the appliance, or that it is not being worn as instructed.

Retention

Remodelling of the supporting tissues continues for some months after tooth movement has been completed. Reitan (1967) has shown that if a tooth is not retained immediately after active movement, tension within the periodontal ligament may be sufficient to reverse the direction of movement for a short period. During the retention period, the periodontal ligament becomes adapted to the new tooth position. At resorption sites, osteoclastic activity ceases and the surface is repaired by the apposition of new bone. At sites of apposition, the loose woven bone, which was laid down during tooth movement, is remodelled and replaced by mature bony trabeculae.

It is sometimes suggested that if the tooth has been moved to a stable position, retention will not be necessary. It is a basic principle of orthodontic treatment that teeth should be moved to positions where long-term stability can be expected. However, unless the tooth movement is held by the occlusion, as when an incisor is moved over the bite, it is normally prudent to retain the tooth with a passive appliance for a period of between 3 and 6 months until the remodelling changes are completed.

Rotations are particularly liable to relapse and over-rotation of the tooth is sometimes recommended, however, this is difficult to achieve with removable appliances. Pericision may be undertaken as a measure to reduce the relapse of rotations (Pinson and Strahan, 1973). Provided that the patient has a good gingival state and it is carefully and skilfully carried out, it is not damaging and is quite effective (Figure 2.9). However, it does not always eliminate relapse. The routine that we recommend for rotations is to carry out pericision and then to retain full time for 6 months followed by at least a year of night-time retention.

References

Christiansen, R.L., Burstone, C.J. (1969) Centres of rotation within the periodontal space. *American Journal of Orthodontics*, **55**: 353–369

Hill, P.A. (1998) Bone remodelling. *British Journal of Orthodontics*, **25**: 101–107

McDonald, F. (1993) Electrical effects at the bone surface. *European Journal of Orthodontics*, **15**: 175–183

Pinson, R.R., Strahan, J.D. (1973) The effect on the relapse of orthodontically rotated teeth of surgical division of the gingival fibres: pericision. *British Journal of Orthodontics*, **1**: 87–92

Reitan, K. (1967) Clinical and histologic observations on tooth movement during and after orthodontic treatment. *American Journal of Orthodontics*, **53**: 721–745

Sandy, J.R., Farndale, R.W., Meikle, M. (1993) Recent advances in understanding mechanically induced bone remodelling and their relevance to orthodontic theory and practice. *American Journal of Orthodontics and Dentofacial Orthopaedics*, **103**: 212–222

Further reading

Yettram, A.L., Wright, K.W.J., Houston, W.J.B. (1977) Centre of rotation of a maxillary central incisor under orthodontic loading. *British Journal of Orthodontics*, **4**: 23–27

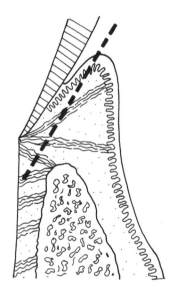

Figure 2.9 Pericision, showing the line of incision to sever the supra-alveolar fibres to reduce rotational relapse.

Chapter 3

Active components

The active components of modern removable appliances comprise springs, bows, screws and elastics. Springs, labial-bows and clasps, made from hard-drawn stainless steel wire, are used most commonly, although when the teeth to be moved are also required for retention of the appliance a screw is preferred (see Figure 9.9, p. 84). Elastics may be used intraorally, or as the active component of headgear.

Stainless steel

When designing, constructing and adjusting springs and bows, it is important to understand some of the basic properties of the material. Stainless steel wire is made by drawing the metal through a series of dies of successively smaller diameter. This process also causes the work-hardening that gives the wire its spring properties. At intervals during the drawing process the wire must be heated to anneal it, otherwise it would become excessively work-hardened and would fracture. The spring properties depend on how much work-hardening has occurred in the final phase. For fixed appliance archwires, high tensile wire may be used, but this is unsuitable for removable appliance components because it is too liable to fracture on bending. Hard drawn wire is the most satisfactory grade.

Stainless steel will be further work-hardened by bending during the construction of components. This can be advantageous in improving spring properties. For example, when a loop is

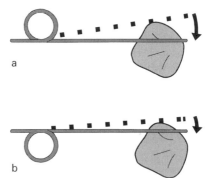

Figure 3.1 (a) A coil spring, which is activated by being 'wound up', is more efficient than a coil spring activated in the opposite direction (b).

bent in a wire, it is differentially stretched so that the outer surface becomes more work-hardened and thus has better spring properties than the inner surface. If the spring is deflected in the same direction as the previous bending, its elastic recovery is better than if it is deflected in the opposite direction (Figure 3.1). This is known as the Bauschinger effect.

Excessive bending will cause sufficient work-hardening to fracture the wire. This is particularly liable to happen if the wire undergoes reverse bending – for example, an incorrect bend which is straightened out is likely to fracture during subsequent use.

Surface damage to the wire during manufacture or, more often, during fabrication or adjustment of a component, also contributes to the possibility of fracture. Surface defects act as 'stress rasors' and provide sites where cracks may start. Problems with wire fracture can be greatly reduced by careful construction and adjustment.

Annealing

A heated wire will eventually reach a temperature at which the grain structure is modified. Stress-relief-annealing occurs between 450 and 500 degrees Celsius. This does not damage the spring properties of the wire (and can sometimes improve them by dissipating induced stresses) but it is generally not considered to be worthwhile for removable appliance components. Heating the wire above 900 degrees Celsius will result in a complete reorganization of the grain structure with loss of the spring properties and this cannot be restored, except by drawing the wire further. Such annealing is liable to occur if the wire is overheated during soldering or welding, so these techniques must be employed carefully and are best used sparingly.

Elgiloy

This is an alloy principally of cobalt and chromium, which can be bent up in the softened state and hardened by heat treating after the bending is completed. It has a greater resistance to stress/strain factor and is used by many operators for construction of Adams' and other clasps, which reduces the likelihood of fracture.

Mechanics of springs

Most orthodontic springs are variants of the simple cantilever. For a round wire, the force generated by a small deflection within its elastic limit depends on the deflection, the cross-sectional area of the wire and the length:

$$F = d*c/l$$

The cross-sectional area of the wire is especially significant. Doubling the wire diameter increases the force 16 times and even using a wire of 0.7 mm rather than 0.5 mm diameter doubles the force for a given deflection. The

ideal spring would have an almost flat load/deflection curve so that the force applied remained almost constant as the tooth moved. For ease of management by the patient the spring should have a reasonably small deflection and should be resistant to displacement and distortion. These criteria cannot all be satisfied simultaneously.

Force

For a single-rooted tooth, a spring should deliver a force in the range of 25–40 g (the lower forces being indicated for teeth with short roots, such as lateral incisors).Very light forces may lie below the threshold for a reasonable rate of tooth movement. Excessive forces delay tooth movement, overload anchorage (Figure 3.2) and may cause discomfort to the patient.

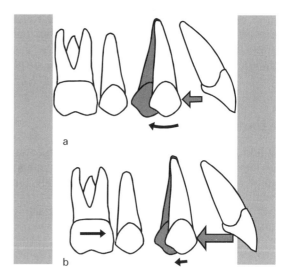

Figure 3.2 The effects of different force values during canine retraction. (a) The correct force produces maximum canine movement and minimum movement of the other teeth. (b) An excessive force may give reduced canine movement and will result in undesirable movement of the other teeth in the arch. An increase in overjet is a sign of this.

Deflection

In most situations, a spring activation of about 3 mm is satisfactory (Figure 3.3). If the spring is given greater activation the patient is more

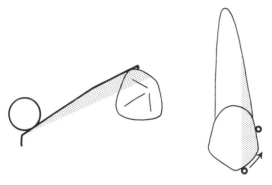

Figure 3.3 Maximum activation of a 0.5 mm palatal canine retraction spring.

ciably less than 1 which means that the spring is less flexible in a mesio-distal direction than it is vertically. This makes them awkward for the operator to adjust and for the patient to manage (Figure 3.4).

Spring design

In order to have maximum flexibility a palatal cantilever spring needs to be as long as possible, however, the dimensions of the oral cavity determine the maximum length of spring. It is usual to incorporate a coil, of about 3 mm

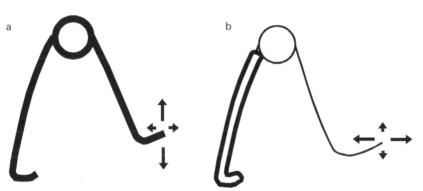

Figure 3.4 Stability ratio of buccal canine springs. (a) The standard buccal canine spring is more flexible vertically than it is mesio-distally. (b) Supported buccal canine retractor has the advantage that it is more flexible mesio-distally than vertically.

likely to insert it incorrectly. With a smaller deflection the force applied will decrease rapidly as the tooth moves so that intermittent movement will have to be accepted unless the spring is activated more frequently. The expected rate of tooth movement is between 1 and 2 mm a month, which means that monthly adjustments are sufficient if an activation of 3 mm is used. The force delivered by palatal springs of 0.5 mm wire increases by about 15 g for each millimetre of deflection, so that an activation of about one-third of a tooth width (3 mm) will deliver a force of about 45 g. If the tooth moves 1 mm in a month, the residual force will be about 30 g, which is still sufficient to produce tooth movement.

Spring stability is also important – the ideal spring should be flexible in the direction of its action but be stiff in other directions, so that it does not readily become displaced. A simple cantilever is equally flexible in all directions and has a stability ratio of 1. This can be improved by support from the baseplate. Some buccal springs have a stability ratio of appre-

internal diameter, in order to increase the effective length of the wire. Whenever possible the coil should be designed so that it 'unwinds' as the tooth moves, because the elastic recovery will be better than that of a spring loaded in the opposite direction. A palatal spring constructed in this manner, which is boxed for protection and made in 0.5 mm wire, has favourable characteristics (Figure 3.5).

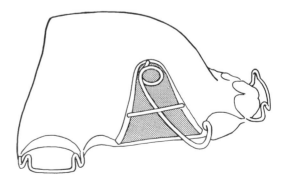

Figure 3.5 A palatal cantilever spring (0.5 mm) boxed and guarded.

Springs are not normally made in wire diameter of less than 0.5 mm, as the patient would readily distort thinner wire and they are not generally recommended.

To give a spring a degree of stability while still retaining flexibility, 0.5 mm wire can be sheathed with stainless steel tubing having an internal diameter of 0.5 mm. The tubing is then incorporated into the acrylic of the appliance. Such supported springs are used for canine retraction and overjet reduction (Figure 3.6).

Unsupported buccal springs (Figure 3.7) and bows have to be made from 0.7 mm wire to provide sufficient strength. Unsupported buccal springs are often rather stiff. Such springs must not be activated by much more than 1 mm, if excessive force is to be avoided. Because the force decays rapidly as the tooth moves, the spring may not remain active throughout the period between visits. This means that continuous tooth movement is difficult to maintain.

Direction of tooth movement

The point of contact between the spring and tooth determines the direction in which the tooth moves. A palatal spring is satisfactory for labial and mesio-distal tooth movements, but a

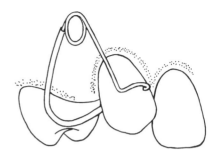

Figure 3.8 A supported buccal canine retractor to move the tooth distally and palatally.

buccal spring must be used if palatal movement is required, or if it is not possible to engage a palatal spring correctly on the tooth surface (Figure 3.8).

Ease of insertion and patient comfort

Most springs are readily managed by the patient but, if palatal finger springs are used to move cheek teeth buccally then correct insertion may be difficult and 'T' springs (Figure 3.9) are preferable. Most palatal springs are comfortable but the ends must be carefully finished to avoid lacerating the patient's buccal mucosa.

Buccal springs and bows can cause discomfort and traumatic ulceration if they have been extended too deeply into the sulcus or if they project buccally, so care must be taken to position such springs correctly when fitting the appliance.

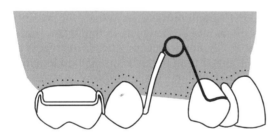

Figure 3.6 A supported buccal canine retractor 0.5 mm wire sheathed in stainless steel tubing.

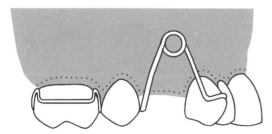

Figure 3.7 Unsupported buccal canine spring 0.7 mm.

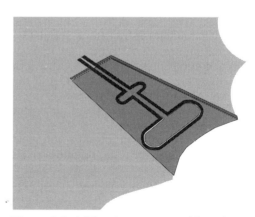

Figure 3.9 A 'T' spring constructed from 0.5 mm wire. Adjustment loops are incorporated so that the spring can be elongated as the tooth moves buccally.

Palatal springs

These springs are used for mesio-distal movement and buccal movement of teeth. They are usually the springs of choice for mesio-distal tooth movement because they are protected by the base plate and so are less liable to damage.

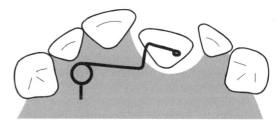

Figure 3.10 A cranked cantilever spring to procline a central incisor.

Single cantilever spring (finger spring)

This spring may be used to move teeth labially or in the line of the arch. It is normally constructed from 0.5 mm hard stainless steel wire. Some operators prefer to use 0.6 mm wire and activate the spring by a smaller amount (50% of the deflection will give about the same force). A coil is incorporated into the spring close to its emergence from the baseplate. This increases the length of wire and thus the flexibility of the spring. For maximal resilience, the coil should lie on the opposite side of the spring from the tooth so that it 'unwinds' as the tooth moves (see Figure 3.1). For labial or buccal movement of teeth, a single cantilever spring should be cranked (Figure 3.10) to keep it clear of the other teeth. This also ensures that the spring is protected by the baseplate even when the tooth moves.

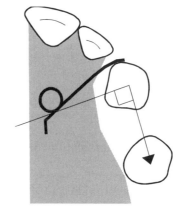

Figure 3.11 The coil of a palatal cantilever spring should lie on a line from the mid-point of the crown at 90 degrees to the direction of movement.

When a palatal cantilever spring is constructed, the intended path of tooth movement is determined and the required point of contact of the spring with the tooth is marked on the model. A line is then drawn on the model, at a right angle to the path of tooth movement and through the mid-crown width of the tooth. This indicates the correct position of the coil (Figure 3.11). The spring arm should be straight unless it has to be cranked to establish the correct contact with the tooth (particularly when it is being used to retract a canine) to ensure that the point of contact with the tooth is correct and that the tooth will move in the right direction (see Figure 2.6, p. 10). The free end is finished neatly after the baseplate has been processed. A palatal spring is usually boxed to protect it from damage, so that it lies in the recess between the baseplate and the mucosa. A possible problem is that if the spring catches between the teeth during removal it may be pulled away from the baseplate. Re-adjustment is difficult and will weaken the spring. If the spring is being used to carry out movement along the line of the arch, such

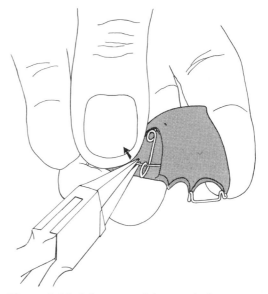

Figure 3.12 Adjustment of the guard wire to ensure free movement of spring.

distortion can be prevented by incorporating a guard wire palatal to it (Figure 3.12) so that a channel is formed between the baseplate and guard. It is important that, during construction, the spring is blocked out adequately, so that it can act freely, and is not impeded by the guard.

The use of a guard is a matter of personal preference and some operators find that guards are more trouble than they are worth. A guard can help to prevent distortion of a spring – which can be difficult to correct – but if the technician does not block out the spring adequately before processing the baseplate, the guard itself may obstruct free movement.

Adjustment

A palatal spring is simple to adjust. Use a dental mirror with the appliance in place to check that the spring contacts the tooth correctly and lies close to the gingival margin (Figure 3.13). At the time of fitting slight activation of no more than 1–2 mm is advisable, but at subsequent visits an adjustment of 3 mm is appropriate. The spring should not be bent where it emerges from the baseplate – this is a site of stress concentration and if the wire is

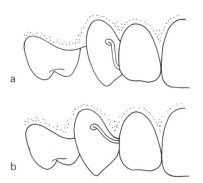

Figure 3.13 (a) When a palatal canine spring is first fitted the spring may have to pass over the contact point between the teeth. (b) Once tooth movement has commenced the spring should be re-contoured closer to the gingival margin.

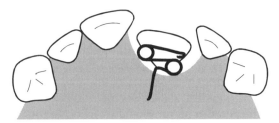

Figure 3.14 A double cantilever spring (0.5 mm wire).

further work-hardened by bending then fracture may occur. The correct site of adjustment is in the free arm of the spring as close to the coil as possible. In cases where the direction of the spring has to be corrected to achieve the intended direction of movement adjustment may be carried out further from the coil.

Double cantilever spring ('Z' spring)

In some situations, particularly where an incisor is to be proclined, space for a single cantilever spring is limited. In these circumstances, a double cantilever, or 'Z' spring (0.5 mm wire) can be used (Figure 3.14). It is important that the limbs are as long as possible, otherwise these springs can be rather stiff. If the limbs of the spring are short, the range of adjustment is limited and the patient may find the appliance difficult to insert. The spring should be perpendicular to the palatal surface of the tooth; otherwise it will tend to slide incisally and to intrude the tooth. If a lateral incisor is to be proclined and space is very short it may be permissible to construct a 'Z' spring in 0.35 mm wire.

The mechanical principles and general features of the double cantilever spring are similar to those of the single cantilever spring.

Adjustment

Adjustment can be carried out to the palatal limb first – close to the coil at the fixed end of the spring to establish the degree of activation – then at the other end of the limb to keep the free limb perpendicular to the intended direction of movement of the tooth. It is often possible to activate the spring in a single movement by grasping its outer arm in the beaks of the pliers and pulling it gently forward and away from the acrylic baseplate.

'T' spring

Where a premolar, or sometimes a canine, is to be moved buccally, the patient may find insertion of the appliance very difficult if a single or double cantilever spring is used. A 'T' spring (see Figure 3.9) made from 0.5 mm wire, can be much simpler to manage. The mechanical principles are similar to those of a single cantilever spring but, as both ends of the spring are incorporated into the acrylic, the flexibility is correspondingly reduced. Fortunately, a large deflection is not indicated in this situation, otherwise the patient may have problems in inserting even this type of spring. It must be recognized that the force applied by the spring has a vertical, as well as a horizontal component. If the tooth surface at the point of contact is nearly vertical (as is usually the case with an upper premolar) the intrusive component is small. If this spring is applied to a sloping surface, such as the cingulum plateau of an upper incisor, the vertical component will be larger and the labial component correspondingly smaller. Even if the 'T' spring initially contacts the more vertical incisal part of the palatal surface of an incisor, it will come to rest on the cingulum plateau as the tooth moves. This reduces the efficiency of the spring and the tooth itself may be intruded. Intrusion is usually unwanted when incisors are to be proclined because stability depends on a positive overbite after treatment. The vertical component also has a displacing effect on the appliance and retention may be a problem. For these reasons, 'T' springs are not usually used for labial movement of upper incisors.

Adjustment

The spring is adjusted by pulling it away from the baseplate. Provided that it is only adjusted by a small amount it should seat itself correctly when the patient inserts the appliance. Once the tooth has moved some distance, it may be necessary to elongate the spring at the adjustment loops.

Coffin spring

This is a strong spring made of a thick gauge wire (1.25 mm) and is used for transverse arch expansion, for example to treat a unilateral crossbite with lateral mandibular displacement (Figure 3.15). It has the advantage over a screw that differential expansion can be obtained in the premolar and molar regions, but the appliance tends to be unstable unless it is expertly made and adjusted. For this reason, a screw may be preferred unless differential expansion of the arch is required.

Adjustment

Before the spring is adjusted, it is useful to drill marking pits in the appliance. Divider readings are taken of the transverse distance between these pits so that the amount of expansion can be controlled. Pliers should not be used to adjust the spring because it is readily distorted. It is safer to expand the appliance by pulling the sides apart manually, first in the premolar and then in the molar regions. Care must be taken to maintain the two sides of the appliance in the same plane during adjustment. If it is twisted vertically, the appliance will not fit and this can be difficult to correct.

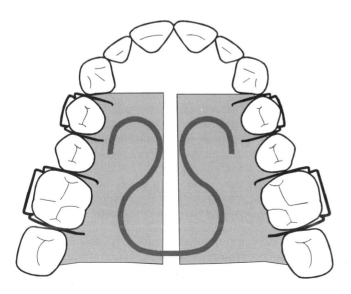

Figure 3.15 A coffin spring (1.25 mm) for transverse arch expansion.

Buccal springs

These springs can be used for mesio-distal tooth movements, palatal tooth movement and, in conjunction with some form of bonded attachment to a tooth, occlusal movement, rotation or buccal movement. Care needs to be taken during construction so that they do not intrude too deeply into the buccal sulcus. Instructing the patient on how to remove the appliance should specifically address the ease with which the buccal springs may be distorted.

Buccal canine retractor

A buccal spring is used where a buccally placed canine has to be moved palatally as well as distally – an operation for which a palatal spring is not satisfactory. Buccal springs are liable to be uncomfortable (which can make

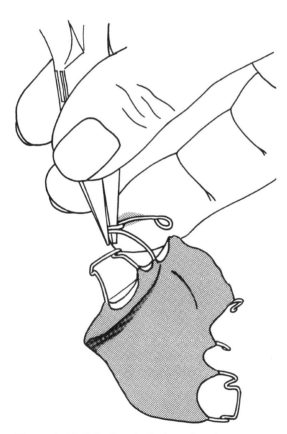

Figure 3.16 Adjustment of a buccal canine retractor.

them unpopular with patients). They are relatively unstable in the vertical dimension (see Figure 3.4) which can make them difficult to adjust, because if the spring acts on a sloping surface, it will tend to slide along the incline. An unsupported buccal spring has to be constructed from 0.7 mm wire to provide stability and will be much less flexible than a palatal spring, so that a small deflection generates a large force.

In view of these problems, particularly careful attention has to be given to the design and construction of a buccal spring. The impression must adequately reproduce the buccal sulcus and show the muscle attachments so that the spring can be kept clear of them. The spring should extend as far as the mucosal reflection and lie just clear of the attached mucosa. The outline of the spring is drawn on the model. The coil lies just distal to the long axis of the tooth, while the anterior limb of the spring passes down from the coil to the middle of the crown and is carried round, in contact with the tooth, to the mesial contact area. This design is more stable, making control of distal and palatal tooth movements simpler than with the conventional buccal retractor (Houston and Waters, 1977). The distal limb of the spring is carried through to the baseplate, in contact with the second premolar and above its contact area.

Adjustment

The spring should be activated by only 1 mm, otherwise the force will be excessive. Provided that it has been constructed to contact the tooth correctly, adjustment is simple. Distal activation is effected at the coil by bending the anterior limb over the round beak of a pair of spring-forming pliers (Figure 3.16). Palatal activation is undertaken in the anterior limb after it emerges from the coil. When the appliance is inserted, the spring may catch on the cuspal incline of the canine and the patient should be instructed to check and correct this if necessary.

Supported buccal retractor

This spring (see Figure 3.6) is identical in design to the buccal retractor described above but is made from 0.5 mm wire supported in tubing. It is more than twice as flexible as the standard retractor, because the shorter free length of wire is more than compensated for by the reduction in diameter. The tubing imparts excellent vertical stability. Although not as flexible as a palatal finger spring, the supported buccal retractor has good mechanical properties and is easy to use, provided that care has been taken to follow the design details.

Adjustment

An activation of 2 mm (about one-quarter of the canine width) is appropriate. It is most important not to bend the wire where it emerges from the tubing, otherwise it may fracture at this site of stress concentration. The adjustment should be made as described for the self-supporting buccal retractor.

Reverse loop buccal retractor

This buccal retractor is favoured by some, particularly where the sulcus is shallow, as in the lower arch (Figure 3.17). Its flexibility depends on the height of the vertical loop, which should be as long as possible. The main problem with this spring is that it is stiff in the horizontal plane yet very unstable vertically. For this reason, in the upper arch, we prefer one of the other buccal retractors.

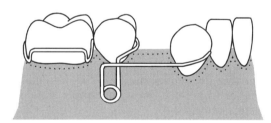

Figure 3.17 A reverse loop buccal canine retractor, 0.7 mm wire.

Adjustment

The spring should be activated by not more than 1 mm. This is most readily done by cutting off 1 mm of wire from the free end and re-forming it to engage the mesial surface of the tooth. Alternatively, it can be activated by opening the loop by 1 mm.

Soldered auxiliary spring

It is possible to solder a spring to the bridge of the Adams' clasp on a first molar (0.6 mm wire or 0.7 mm wire). Two versions are available. The spring can be used to tuck an outstanding canine or premolar into line during the final stages of treatment (Figure 3.18).

Advantages

The spring does not cross the embrasure and so does not compete with other wirework. (As a general principle it is sensible to avoid taking two wires through a single embrasure.) The spring can be added easily to an existing appliance and, if necessary, may be cranked to correct an outstanding canine through the loop of the labial bow on a retainer. The length – and hence the flexibility of the spring – can be controlled by the choice of an appropriate wire size and where necessary by bringing the wire from the distal end of the bridge of the clasp and recurving it forwards (Figure 3.18). (This may be particularly useful when a second premolar has to be moved palatally.)

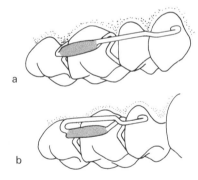

Figure 3.18 A soldered auxiliary spring (0.7 mm wire). (a) To move a canine palatally. (b) A re-curved spring to move a premolar palatally.

Disadvantages

A certain level of expertise with solder is required if the spring is to be attached satisfactorily without annealing the wire of the clasp. When the clasp is adjusted the spring position is also affected and may require compensatory adjustment. It is also difficult to add this spring to a clasp that is already carrying a soldered tube for the application of a facebow.

Bows

Bows may be active or passive and will usually span a number of teeth. Both ends of the bow are incorporated in the acrylic. Active bows are used for incisor retraction. The bow selected will depend partly on the preference of the operator and partly on the amount of retraction required. Flexible bows, such as the Roberts' retractor, are most suitable where a large overjet has to be reduced. When the amount of retraction is small but minor irregularities need to be corrected (and perhaps over-corrected) a less flexible bow may be preferred because it is more precise in its action and needs only a small amount of activation.

Roberts' retractor

This is a flexible bow that is constructed from 0.5 mm diameter wire inserted into stainless steel tubing to give support at either end of the bow (Figure 3.19). A coil is placed at the point of emergence of the wire from the tubing. The tubing emerges from the baseplate distal to the canines. The horizontal section of the bow is bent into the smooth curve to which the incisors should conform. Even if the incisors are irregular, the curve of the bow should be smooth and they will be gathered in as they are retracted. A common fault is to make this horizontal section too short so that it fails to control the lateral incisors. The flexibility of this bow lies in the vertical limbs and coils that should be of adequate size (at least 3 mm in internal diameter).

Adjustment

This bow is light and flexible. An adjustment of about 3 mm is suitable but the site of adjustment is very important because if the wire is bent where it emerges from the supporting tube (a site of stress concentration) it will often fracture. The bow is adjusted by bending it in the vertical limb below the coil. Provided that the spring has been carefully made and adjusted correctly, fracture is rare. As the incisors move palatally, the bow will drop anteriorly and the level of the horizontal part will have to be adjusted.

High labial bow with apron spring

In concept, this is similar to the Roberts' retractor. A heavy base arch of 0.9 mm wire extends into the buccal sulcus (Figure 3.20). The impression must be muscle-trimmed so that the buccal and labial fraenae can be avoided. There is no need to extend the base arch to the full depth of the sulcus because the apron spring is very flexible. When the baseplate is to be cold-cured, it is simplest to attach the apron spring before the appliance is processed, but where the appliance has to be flasked for a heat-cured baseplate, the apron spring should be attached after the baseplate is processed. The apron spring (0.35–0.4 mm) is attached to the base arch by wrapping a few turns round the vertical step and the active spring is formed by two or three turns around the horizontal part. After the apron has been formed, its free end is attached to the base arch in the manner already described for the fixed end. Practice is required before an apron spring can be neatly formed and it is necessary to use an adequate length of wire and to maintain it under steady tension as it is wound on to the base arch. After the appliance has been finished, the base arch may be made more comfortable for the patient by removing the central portion. This also makes it easier to replace the apron spring should it fracture during use.

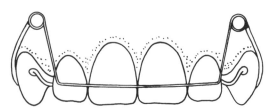

Figure 3.19 A Roberts' retractor made from 0.5 mm wire supported in tubing of 0.5 mm internal diameter.

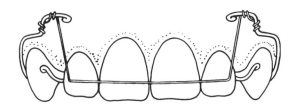

Figure 3.20 A high labial bow (0.9 mm) with an apron spring (0.4 mm). The central portion of the high labial bow is removed after the baseplate has been processed.

The apron spring has good mechanical properties but the Roberts' retractor is simpler to construct and more comfortable for the patient which makes it preferable. Some orthodontists use the high labial arch with apron spring because repair is possible at the chairside but rewinding an apron spring can be tedious and, given the precautions outlined above, the Roberts' retractor will give little trouble.

Adjustment

The bow is adjusted in the vertical limb as described for the Roberts' retractor.

Labial bow with 'U' loops

This is constructed on 0.7 mm wire. Flexibility depends largely on the vertical height of the loops (Figure 3.21). Sulcus depth is limited, however, and because the wire is heavy these bows are very rigid in the horizontal plane. Conversely, they are flexible in a vertical

direction and so the stability ratio is poor. Minor movements of individual teeth can be obtained by incorporating bayonet bends at appropriate points (Figure 3.22). The major advantage of the labial bow with 'U' loops is that if only minor overjet reduction or incisor alignment is required, it may be incorporated into an appliance with palatal springs for canine retraction. When the canines are retracted sufficiently, the bow may be adjusted to retract the incisors. In view of the heavy forces generated by very minor activation of these bows, with the associated risk of anchorage loss, it is better to modify the bow for incisor retraction as described below. *Note*: If the overjet is greater than 4 mm, it is usually wiser to use a second appliance with a more flexible bow.

Adjustment

To reduce an overjet, the bow is adjusted at the 'U' loops. This adjustment must be small. The bow should be displaced palatally by only 1 mm. The flexibility can be greatly increased by dividing the labial bow at the incisor retraction stage, so that there are two buccal arms (Figure 3.23). This split bow is quite suitable for incisor retraction but care must be taken during adjustment to preserve the correct curve and not to flatten off the arch anteriorly. This is achieved by adjusting the bow at the 'U' loops, rather than in the horizontal arms. Rotations or minor individual tooth movements are difficult to control with a split bow.

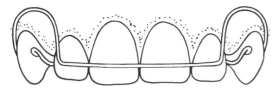

Figure 3.21 A 'U' loop labial bow (0.7 mm) with passive stops mesial to the canines.

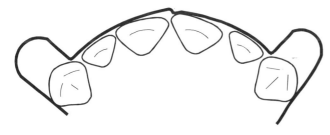

Figure 3.22 A bayonet bend for minor adjustment of incisor position.

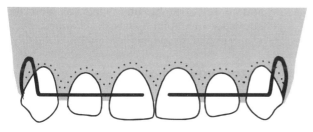

Figure 3.23 Flexibility of a 'U' loop labial bow is greatly increased if it is divided.

a

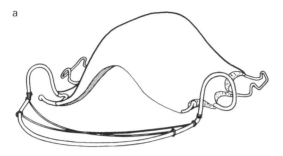

b

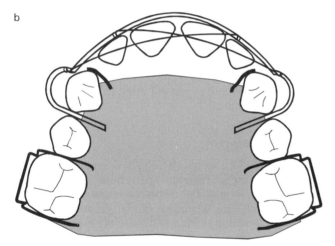

Figure 3.24 Self-straightening wires (0.5 mm) on a labial bow (0.7 mm). Self-straightening wires are wound loosely on to the bow so that they can slide freely along it. (a) A labial view. (b) A palatal view showing the self-straightening wires in their passive position.

Self-straightening wires

A modification of a labial bow to increase its flexibility can be made by adding a self-straightening wire, which can be used to reduce an overjet (Figure 3.24). Individual tooth movements cannot be undertaken and there is a tendency for this device to flatten the arch anteriorly, although the use of two wires will minimize this tendency.

Adjustment

This is done by closing the 'U' loops of the bow and adjusting its level as necessary. Care must be taken to ensure that self-straightening wires run freely on the supporting bow.

Labial bow with reverse loops

This is similar to the bow described above except that reverse loops are used (Figure 3.25). These loops must be well clear of the clasps on the first molars or they will be difficult to adjust. It is sometimes claimed that this type of bow will prevent buccal drift of the canines during their retraction, but the primary method of controlling canine movement should be by correct adjustment of the spring, rather than by relying on the bow to compensate for careless adjustment. This bow is rather rigid and should be activated by only 1 mm at any time.

Adjustment

The adjustment is carried out in two stages (Figure 3.26). The vertical loop is first opened by compressing it with pliers. This lowers the bow in the incisor region so that compensating bends must be made at the base of the loops. The flexibility of the bow with reverse loops can be improved either by dividing it or by adding self-straightening wires, as described above for the labial bow with 'U' loops.

Extended labial bow

This labial bow is also made from 0.7 mm wire but its flexibility is greatly increased by the

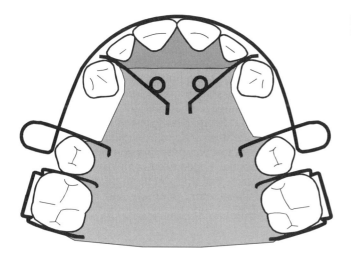

Figure 3.25 A reverse loop labial bow (0.7 mm).

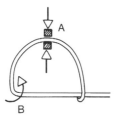

Figure 3.26 Adjustment of a reverse loop labial bow. When the pliers compress the loop at A, the anterior part of the bow drops down and a compensating bend needs to be made at B.

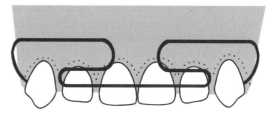

Figure 3.27 An extended labial bow (0.7 mm).

enlarged loops (Figure 3.27). This bow is a useful alternative to the Roberts' retractor for reduction of an overjet and it is also suitable for the alignment of irregular incisors. Due to the size of the loops, it may be less comfortable for the patient to wear.

Adjustment

The bow must be adjusted with care to avoid trauma to the buccal mucosa.

Screws

An alternative method of providing a force is to use a screw as an integral part of the removable appliance. The screw normally transmits its force by means of the acrylic, which comes in contact with the teeth. The patient usually activates a screw once or twice a week. A fairly high force is generated but is intermittent.

Nevertheless, there are certain situations in which screws are very useful.

Many types of screw are commercially available for use in removable appliances. Desirable features in a screw are adequate travel, stability and minimal bulk (Haynes and Jackson, 1962). Screws can be used for many tooth movements, but they add to the expense of an appliance while making it more bulky. Adjustment is normally carried out once or twice weekly by the patient. We recommend screws only in those few situations where springs would be unsatisfactory: for example, where the teeth to be moved are required for retention of the appliance (see Figure 9.9 p. 84). Single and double guide pin screws are available (Figure 3.28). The latter are more stable but the former is useful where space is limited. Problems can occur with screws. Some tend to turn back under load. If the appliance is left out it may not be possible for the patient to re-insert it and treatment may thus be

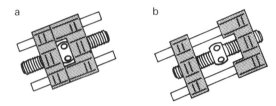

Figure 3.28 A double guide pin screw. (a) Closed. (b) Open.

delayed. Screws apply intermittent large forces, which decrease as tooth movement occurs. The large force is acceptable only because the activation at any one time is small (less than 0.2 mm). The tooth is thus moved within the limits of the periodontal ligament and extensive hyalinization will not be produced. Spring-loaded screws are available, in which a spring within the screw dissipates the force over a period of time. Although these offer theoretical advantages, they are bulkier, more expensive and seem to offer few clinical advantages.

Adjustment

The patient is given the key to adjust the screw. It is worthwhile incorporating a marker in the baseplate to indicate the direction in which the screw is to be turned. An adjustment of one quarter-turn each week will produce a rate of tooth movement of about 1 mm per month. The patient must ensure that the appliance seats home fully after adjustment. In some situations it is possible to adjust the screw twice weekly, but this may lead to anchorage loss and the appliance may not seat home fully, so that retention is less good. It is possible to monitor the expansion achieved by the use of holes drilled into the acrylic in each half of appliance and to measure with dividers at each visit. Alternatively the screw may be turned back at each visit and the number of turns recorded in the notes.

Elastics

Elastics may be used intraorally with removable appliances and may be particularly useful in conjunction with a bonded attachment to produce localized tooth movement. They can also be used, as described below, to provide intermaxillary traction.

To align a displaced tooth, a point of attachment needs to be bonded to the tooth – usually a stainless steel hook or button. An elastic can then be engaged between the appliance and the displaced tooth. Elastics need to be changed by the patient on a regular basis and care must be used not to exceed the appropriate force limits. Elastics have been used in an attempt to reduce an overjet, but this is generally considered to be an unsatisfactory method and is not recommended.

Intermaxillary traction

A removable appliance may be fitted in the opposing arch to a fixed appliance, to allow the use of intermaxillary elastics. This is particularly useful when there is a well-aligned lower arch, which does not require any active tooth movement. A well fitting removable appliance can provide an anchorage point for either class II or class III elastic traction. The use of elastic intermaxillary traction with removable appliances alone is not satisfactory.

Localized tooth movement

Intraoral elastics can be used to move a single tooth. A hook, bonded on to the surface of the tooth provides a point of attachment for the elastic, which also engages an appropriately placed hook on the appliance.

Occlusal movement of partially erupted teeth can be satisfactorily achieved by this method and the palatal acrylic of the appliance provides anchorage for the movement.

Buccally placed canines that are crowded and partially erupted can also be retracted in this manner. The hook can be bonded on to the buccal surface of the tooth. The removable appliance carries a buccal arm with a hook at the end of the arm, which is positioned so that it is possible to apply an occlusally directed force on the tooth. The patient has to engage the elastic when fitting the appliance and a certain degree of manual dexterity is necessary. Teeth that are erupting palatally are considerably more difficult for a patient to engage with an elastic and may be better brought into the arch with full fixed appliances.

Elastics have been used to carry out the retraction of incisors. A latex elastic is stretched between hooks placed distal to the canines and provides an inconspicuous method of retracting incisors. A serious drawback is that the elastic is liable to slide up the teeth and traumatize the gingivae. This can be prevented by bonding a plastic bracket to the labial surface of a central incisor but, because elastics also tend to flatten the arch, they are generally better avoided for overjet reduction with removable appliances.

References

Haynes, S., Jackson, D. (1962) A comparison of the mechanism and efficiency of twenty-one orthodontic expansion screws. *Dental Practitioner*, **13**: 125–133

Houston, W.J.B., Waters, N.E. (1977) The design of buccal canine retraction springs for removable orthodontic appliances. *British Journal of Orthodontics*, **4**: 191–195

Further reading

Houston, W.J.B., Waters, N.E., Farrant, S.D. (1972) High tensile wires and removable appliances. *British Journal of Orthodontics*, **1**: 33–36

Muir, J.D. (1971) Anterior retention in the removable appliance. *Transactions of the BSSO*, **57**: 178–184

Chapter 4

Appliance retention

The term 'retention' can have two completely different meanings within orthodontics. It is used to describe the support that is given to the teeth after a period of orthodontic treatment in order to maintain their improved alignment and relationship. In the field of removable appliances the same term is also used to describe the resistance of the appliance to displacement. This chapter is concerned with the *retention of the appliance in the mouth*. Chapter 11 covers the use of removable appliances as retainers.

Appliance retention is provided by wires, in the form of clasps and bows. Good retention is essential if treatment is to proceed efficiently and needs to be planned carefully. This is particularly important if headgear is to be worn with the appliance. Even where retention is good it is prudent to reduce to a minimum any forces that tend to displace the appliance. Examples of such forces might be springs acting on cuspal inclines, extraoral force applied in a downward direction, or rocking of the appliance due to contact of the lower incisors upon an excessively undercut anterior bite plane. The patient will find it harder to tolerate an appliance that is not a firm fit and progress is likely to suffer.

When removable appliances were first used, clasping was a particular problem. The arrowhead clasp was one of the most successful designs but was awkward to make and to adjust. The arrowhead engages the embrasure between teeth but, although this can offer good retention, it is easy to damage the gingival papillae and the adjacent teeth can be sepa-rated by the action of the clasp. The design by Adams (1955) of the modified arrowhead clasp now known as the Adams' clasp represented a major advance in removable appliance retention.

Posterior retention

The Adams' clasp (Figure 4.1)

This clasp, like most others, is made from 0.7 mm stainless steel wire or from Elgiloy (although for clasps on deciduous teeth 0.6 mm wire is more suitable). It engages the mesio-buccal and disto-buccal undercuts that can be found on the crown of almost every tooth. A depth of undercut of about 0.25 mm is ideal.

In children, where the anatomical crowns of the teeth may not be fully exposed, undercuts may be difficult to locate, but they can generally be found at the mesio-buccal and disto-buccal

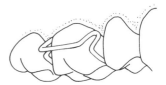

Figure 4.1 An Adams' clasp (0.7 mm wire). The clasp engages undercuts on the mesio-buccal and disto-buccal aspects of the tooth. The bridge stands clear of the buccal surface and the wire is closely adapted to the tooth where it passes across the contact area.

aspects of the crown just below the gingival margin. The model must be carefully trimmed to reproduce the anatomical contour of the crown so that when the appliance is constructed, the clasps engage the undercuts snugly. Overzealous trimming of the model will make the appliance impossible to insert without extensive adjustment. Too little trimming may mean that retention is inadequate and there may be little prospect of improving it subsequently.

In adults the opposite problem can occur. Undercuts at the gingival margin may be too deep, particularly if there has been gingival recession. Clasps are too stiff to engage deep undercuts and, if they are made to do so, the appliance will be impossible to insert. Adjustment of the clasps to allow the appliance to be fitted means that they do not contact the tooth surface and so the appliance will be loose, with little prospect of satisfactory modification. In such cases the clasps must only engage the required depth of undercut and should not extend as far as the gingival margin.

Advantages of the Adams' clasp

The advantages of the Adams' clasp are as follows:

- Its bridge provides a site to which the patient can apply pressure with the fingertips during removal of the appliance
- Auxiliary springs can be soldered to the bridge of the clasp
- Hooks can be soldered to the clasp or bent in during its construction to accept intermaxillary traction
- Tubes can be soldered to the bridge of the clasp to accommodate a facebow for extra-oral traction.

Soldering must be carefully carried out, since the use of excess heat can lead to softening of the wire, which will reduce the efficiency of the clasp.

Adjustment of the Adams' clasp

Construction of the Adams' clasp is not simple (see Appendix 1), but the clasp is effective and can be readily adjusted at the chairside (see Figure 10.7, p. 90). When the appliance is seated a clasp should be nearly passive. Active clasps can exert a palatal force on the teeth, so that if the appliance does not seat fully they will tend to be tipped under the baseplate, so reduc-

ing the depth of the undercut. A vicious circle can then occur as further tightening, in an attempt to improve retention, produces further tooth movement, which makes the situation worse. It is even possible to create a crossbite, which can only be corrected by the use of an additional appliance. Such problems are liable to occur where retention was initially poor due to faulty appliance design and construction, sometimes compounded by an awkward crown form. It can be avoided only by careful scrutiny and trimming of the model, thoughtful clasp placement and careful routine adjustment.

Lower molars

In some cases, lower molars have little available undercut on the buccal surface and consequently retention of a lower appliance may not be satisfactory. Adjustment of the clasp to try to increase the retention may result in an appliance that does not seat satisfactorily. One solution to the problem of lack of buccal undercut on lower molars is to use an appliance with clasping on the lingual side (see below).

Variants of the Adams' clasp

Adams described variations of this clasp (Figure 4.2) suited to most teeth, deciduous and permanent. Soldered auxiliary clasps that utilize further undercuts are seldom used, as they are awkward to adjust. An alternative is to add an accessory spur made from 0.8 mm wire with a single arrowhead closed to provide a smooth end (Figure 4.3).

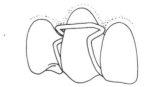

Figure 4.2 An Adams' clasp (0.6 mm wire) on a canine.

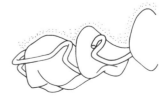

Figure 4.3 A single arrowhead (0.8 mm wire).

Limitations

The Adams' clasp has few limitations but, if it is not skilfully made and adjusted, the wire may become excessively work-hardened and will be liable to fracture. Fracture at the arrowhead can sometimes be repaired by soldering. The other common site of fracture is where the wire passes across the occlusion and, should this occur, it is best to replace the clasp. Some patients find the bridge irritating, particularly if it is too prominent. This most often happens where tubes for headgear are soldered to molar clasps.

The Jackson clasp

The Jackson clasp passes around the gingival margin of the molar (Figure 4.4). It may be conveniently used for deciduous molars using 0.6 mm wire.

Buccal acrylic lower appliances

To overcome the problem of limited undercut on the buccal aspect of lower molars, appliances have been described with clasping on the lingual aspect of the molars (Bell, 1983). Two acrylic baseplates are used, one on each side resting on the buccal mucosa. The acrylic is connected across the anterior labial mucosa by a stainless steel bar. A modified Jackson clasp is used on the lingual aspect engaging the lingual undercuts of the molars (Figure 4.5). The main use of such an appliance is to retract mesially inclined lower canines.

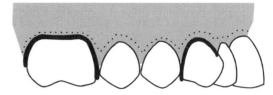

Figure 4.4 The Jackson clasp (0.7 mm wire) on an upper first molar. A recurved clasp used on a canine (0.6 mm wire).

Anterior retention

The Adams' clasp

The Adams' clasp can be used to provide retention at the front of the arch and commonly a double clasp is used spanning both central incisors (Figure 4.6). Alternatively, a clasp may be used on a single incisor. The Adams' clasp is most suited to situations where the central incisors are upright or only mildly proclined. When there is no anterior spacing, the arm of the clasp will pass over the top of the embrasure between the central and lateral incisors. The clasp is prone to breakage where it crosses the embrasure.

A double incisor clasp can be uncomfortable for the patient and where the incisors are very proclined the clasp has to be placed fairly close to the incisor edge to avoid an excessive undercut. It is possible to modify the clasp by curving the bridge and flattening the arrowhead so it is less prominent (Figure 4.7).

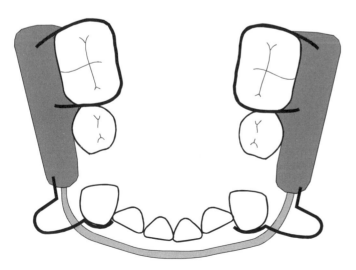

Figure 4.5 A lower appliance with buccal acrylic and lingually placed molar clasps. The buccal acrylic is connected anteriorly by a stainless steel bar.

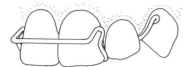

Figure 4.6 A double Adams' clasp (0.7 mm wire). The position of the arrowheads is determined by the depth of the undercuts. Frequently the arrowheads do not need to reach the gingival margin.

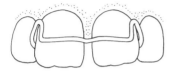

Figure 4.7 A modified double Adams' incisor clasp with the bridge adapted to the labial surfaces of the central incisors.

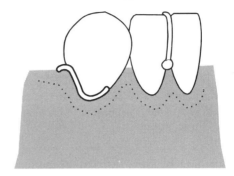

Figure 4.8 A ball ended clasp between the lower incisors engaging the embrasure undercut. A recurved clasp is shown on the lower canine.

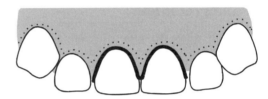

Figure 4.9 The Southend clasp (0.7 mm wire).

The ball-ended clasp

This uses the undercut provided by the embrasure and provides effective retention. The use of the embrasure is not generally desirable because of the danger of gingival damage and tooth separation, but the clasp may occasionally be of use when deciduous teeth must be used for retention (Figure 4.8).

The recurved clasp

This simple clasp uses the same undercuts, as does the Adams' clasp. It is simpler to construct but less effective than the latter and does not allow the attachment of auxiliary components such as headgear tubes (Figure 4.8).

The Southend clasp

The Southend clasp is easy to construct, unobtrusive and well tolerated. The wire passes round the gingival margin of the central incisors and engages undercut between the incisors (Stephens, 1979). It is the preferred anterior clasp, particularly if the incisors are proclined and can be modified to fit between a central and lateral incisor. Breakage is relatively uncommon (Figure 4.9).

The fitted labial bow

This offers good retention on proclined upper incisors but it is less satisfactory on upright teeth. A short bow can fit over both central incisors (Figure 4.10), but more commonly the bow fits over the central and lateral incisors (Figure 4.11). Where the incisors are very

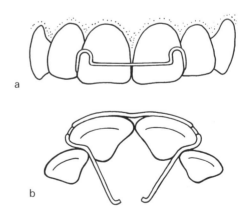

a

b

Figure 4.10 A short fitted labial bow on upper central incisors (0.7 mm wire). This design permits some drifting of the lateral incisors as the canines are retracted.

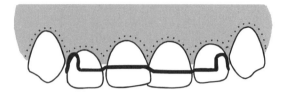

Figure 4.11 A fitted labial bow (0.7 mm wire).

proclined, a labial bow fitted to the incisor third of the crowns may give an easier path of insertion of the appliance.

Planning retention

The positioning of retentive components is important and must be planned for each individual appliance, taking into account the forces that will tend to produce displacement. It is unwise to attempt to clasp every available tooth because this may make the appliance difficult for the patient to manage – as well as making adjustment complicated and interfering with tooth movement. For a simple 'retainer',

Adams' clasps on the upper first molars may give adequate retention, but for an active appliance three or four point retention is generally advisable (Muir, 1971). During canine retraction, for example, a Southend clasp on the upper central incisors may supplement the molar clasps to give good retention. Where a molar is being moved distally with a screw, or where an incisor is being proclined, additional clasps on one or both first premolars may offer a way of producing excellent retention. Retention need not be symmetrical but can be tailored to suit the task of the particular appliance.

References

Adams, C.P. (1955) *The design and construction of removable orthodontic appliances*. John Wright and Sons Ltd, Bristol

Bell, C. (1983) A modified lower removable appliance using lingual clasping and soft tissue anchorage. *British Journal of Orthodontics*, **10**: 162–163

Muir, J.D. (1971) Anterior retention in the removable appliance. *Transactions of the BSSO*, **57**: 178–184

Stephens, C.D. (1979) The Southend clasp. *British Journal of Orthodontics*, **6**: 183–184

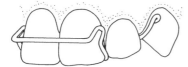

Figure 4.6 A double Adams' clasp (0.7 mm wire). The position of the arrowheads is determined by the depth of the undercuts. Frequently the arrowheads do not need to reach the gingival margin.

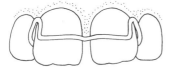

Figure 4.7 A modified double Adams' incisor clasp with the bridge adapted to the labial surfaces of the central incisors.

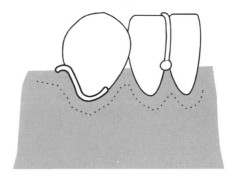

Figure 4.8 A ball ended clasp between the lower incisors engaging the embrasure undercut. A recurved clasp is shown on the lower canine.

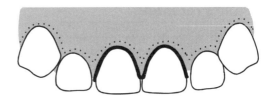

Figure 4.9 The Southend clasp (0.7 mm wire).

The ball-ended clasp

This uses the undercut provided by the embrasure and provides effective retention. The use of the embrasure is not generally desirable because of the danger of gingival damage and tooth separation, but the clasp may occasionally be of use when deciduous teeth must be used for retention (Figure 4.8).

The recurved clasp

This simple clasp uses the same undercuts, as does the Adams' clasp. It is simpler to construct but less effective than the latter and does not allow the attachment of auxiliary components such as headgear tubes (Figure 4.8).

The Southend clasp

The Southend clasp is easy to construct, unobtrusive and well tolerated. The wire passes round the gingival margin of the central incisors and engages undercut between the incisors (Stephens, 1979). It is the preferred anterior clasp, particularly if the incisors are proclined and can be modified to fit between a central and lateral incisor. Breakage is relatively uncommon (Figure 4.9).

The fitted labial bow

This offers good retention on proclined upper incisors but it is less satisfactory on upright teeth. A short bow can fit over both central incisors (Figure 4.10), but more commonly the bow fits over the central and lateral incisors (Figure 4.11). Where the incisors are very

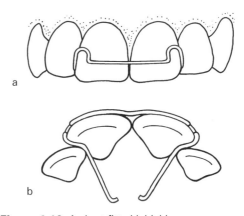

Figure 4.10 A short fitted labial bow on upper central incisors (0.7 mm wire). This design permits some drifting of the lateral incisors as the canines are retracted.

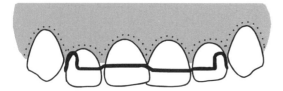

Figure 4.11 A fitted labial bow (0.7 mm wire).

proclined, a labial bow fitted to the incisor third of the crowns may give an easier path of insertion of the appliance.

Planning retention

The positioning of retentive components is important and must be planned for each individual appliance, taking into account the forces that will tend to produce displacement. It is unwise to attempt to clasp every available tooth because this may make the appliance difficult for the patient to manage – as well as making adjustment complicated and interfering with tooth movement. For a simple 'retainer',

Adams' clasps on the upper first molars may give adequate retention, but for an active appliance three or four point retention is generally advisable (Muir, 1971). During canine retraction, for example, a Southend clasp on the upper central incisors may supplement the molar clasps to give good retention. Where a molar is being moved distally with a screw, or where an incisor is being proclined, additional clasps on one or both first premolars may offer a way of producing excellent retention. Retention need not be symmetrical but can be tailored to suit the task of the particular appliance.

References

Adams, C.P. (1955) *The design and construction of removable orthodontic appliances*. John Wright and Sons Ltd, Bristol

Bell, C. (1983) A modified lower removable appliance using lingual clasping and soft tissue anchorage. *British Journal of Orthodontics*, **10**: 162–163

Muir, J.D. (1971) Anterior retention in the removable appliance. *Transactions of the BSSO*, **57**: 178–184

Stephens, C.D. (1979) The Southend clasp. *British Journal of Orthodontics*, **6**: 183–184

Chapter 5

The baseplate

The acrylic baseplate constitutes the body of the removable appliance. It has three functions: it provides a foundation, which supports other components such as springs and clasps; it contributes to anchorage through its contact with the palatal vault and teeth that are not being moved; and it may be built up into bite planes to disengage the occlusion or produce overbite reduction.

Design and construction

The baseplate needs to be thick enough to carry the retentive and active components, but should be as thin as possible, compatible with strength. Ideally, this should be about as thick as a sheet of modelling wax. Thicker appliances may be tolerated but, particularly initially, may be difficult for the patient to wear. The baseplate should normally cover most of the hard palate, finishing just distal to the first molars. It should fit closely around the necks of teeth that are not being moved – otherwise food packing and gingival hyperplasia may occur. It should be trimmed well clear of the teeth to be moved and care must be taken during manufacture to position wire tags in the acrylic so that trimming is possible.

During appliance construction undercuts rarely present a problem in young patients but, for adults, undercuts may require blocking out before the appliance is made. When lower appliances are used undercuts regularly require blocking out.

Acrylic

Orthodontic appliance baseplates are generally manufactured from cold-cured acrylic. It is economical in terms of laboratory-time and warpage is less than with heat-cured acrylic. It does, however, have more free monomer present after curing and the appliance is less strong. The extra expense of a heat-cured appliance may be justified where breakage is liable to be a problem. Examples might be the presence of a deep overbite and very heavy occlusal forces, the need for shallow but strong posterior bite planes and the situation in which a prosthetic tooth must be added to an orthodontic appliance.

Anchorage considerations

In order to obtain maximum anchorage the acrylic should cover most of the palatal mucosa, finishing distal to the first molars, although it may include the second molars if they have erupted fully. The acrylic should contact all the teeth in the arch with the exception of those that will be moved. Where screws are to be used, consideration must be given to the position of the split of the appliance and its influence on the number of teeth to be moved. Where equal movement of groups of teeth is required, for example upper arch expansion, the split should be along the mid-line with equal contact to similar groups of teeth. Where unilateral distal movement is necessary,

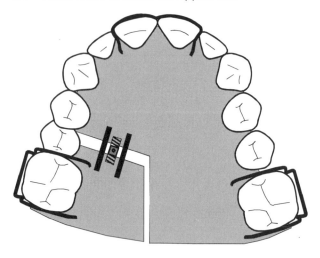

Figure 5.1 An appliance to move a first molar distally. To achieve maximum anchorage, the larger section of the base plate contacts the palate and all the teeth that are not being moved.

however, the appliance should be split to take into account the relative anchorage balance of the number of teeth to be moved and the teeth required to resist the movement. If minimum movement in the anchorage teeth is desired, the maximum number of anchorage teeth should be in contact with the acrylic of the appliance (Figure 5.1).

Bite planes

The acrylic of the baseplate may be thickened anteriorly to provide an anterior bite plane or extended to cover the posterior teeth to form a posterior bite plane. Careful thought about the design and construction of a bite plane can save considerable chairside time later.

Anterior bite plane

The principal use of anterior bite planes is in the reduction of overbite. This occurs primarily by alteration in the rate of eruption of the posterior teeth relative to the eruption of the lower incisors that are in contact with the bite plane. Overbite reduction by this method is most successful in an actively growing patient. In an adult, overbite reduction can sometimes be successfully achieved using a biteplate, but the amount of overbite reduction that can be obtained is less than that for a child patient, takes time to achieve and may not remain stable.

When designing an appliance which includes an anterior bite plane, it is best to specify to the laboratory the overjet and the desired height of the bite plane relative to the palate and the palatal surface of the upper incisors. This enables the laboratory to construct the bite-plate to the correct size. The posterior limit of the bite plane should extend just sufficiently to engage the lower incisors and, ideally, the laboratory should have the study models available to check this dimension (Figure 5.2). Bite planes should be made with the occlusal surface parallel to the occlusal plane. Inclined bite planes may sometimes be required, but may cause proclination of the lower labial segment, which is usually an undesirable tooth movement.

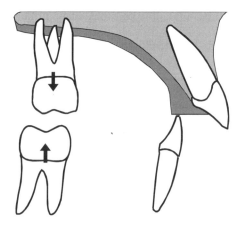

Figure 5.2 An anterior bite plane to reduce the overbite by allowing vertical development of the posterior teeth. The bite plane should be thick enough to separate the posterior teeth by 2–3 mm and extend sufficiently to engage the lower incisors when the mandible is retruded.

When anterior bite planes are used in adults, the initial bite plane should be very thin, because it is often more difficult for an adult to tolerate the same degree of bite opening as a younger patient.

Posterior bite plane

Posterior bite planes can be used to eliminate a lateral or anterior displacement of the mandible. Posterior bite planes will assist in the correction of a buccal crossbite or an anterior crossbite by preventing interference by the opposing teeth and allowing the mandible to adopt a centric position (Figure 5.3).

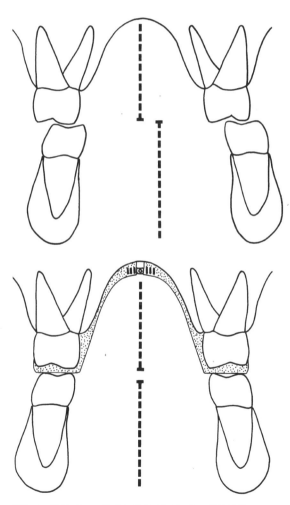

Figure 5.3 A posterior bite plane. A unilateral crossbite may be corrected by arch expansion. Posterior bite planes are incorporated to free the occlusion and eliminate any associated displacing activity.

Posterior bite planes need to be thinner posteriorly than anteriorly and should contact the opposing teeth on both sides of the mouth. They are difficult to construct accurately unless the models have been set up on an articulator. If this is done in the laboratory then considerable time will be saved at the fitting appointment.

Adjustments to the acrylic

Initial fitting of the appliance

Removable appliances should ideally be fitted within 2 weeks of the impressions being taken. Provided that no tooth movement has occurred in the meantime, the baseplate should fit without adjustment. If this is not the case any trimming should be done with care and should be carried out from the fitting surface, because small gaps between the baseplate and the teeth encourage food packing.

If there is any difficulty in seating the appliance it may be best to bend the clasps gently away from the teeth to check whether the resistance is from the baseplate or from the wires. If there are undercuts, the acrylic should be carefully trimmed from them without touching the edge of the polished surface of the appliance so that this still contacts the teeth.

Once the appliance can be fitted, it should be examined in the mouth to ensure that the acrylic is clear of the teeth that are to be moved. The appliance should be removed and retried if necessary to ensure that there is no interference with the intended movement and that gingival hyperplasia will not be encouraged.

Anterior bite planes

Anterior bite planes should be horizontal transversely and anteroposteriorly, so that when the appliance is in place the premolars are separated by 2 or 3 mm. Ideally the bite plane should be flat but, if the lower incisors are irregular, it may be necessary to adjust it to contact at least three of them. As overbite reduction occurs the bite plane can be built up and levelled with the addition of cold-cured acrylic. Overbite reduction should be evident within the first 2 months of fitting the appliance. Some clinicians will build up the bite plane by a small amount every few visits as long as overbite reduction is needed. Most children, however, can tolerate a greater opening and this means that greater increments can be added less frequently. If the bite plane is constructed to half the incisor height on the first appliance and to full incisor height on the second, few, if any, chairside increments will be required. It is wise to wait until the posterior teeth have regained contact before undermining the bite plane to permit overjet reduction. In adults, overbite reduction is difficult to achieve and will take place slowly, so it is important to increase the thickness of the bite plane slowly with progressive additions of cold-cured acrylic as the overbite reduces.

Anterior bite plane adjustment and overjet reduction

Before the upper incisors can be retracted to reduce an overjet the anterior bite plane will need to be trimmed away from these teeth. It will also require later progressive, careful reduction so that the lower incisors maintain their contact with it until the overjet is almost corrected. These teeth will otherwise re-erupt and the overbite increase again. The acrylic should first be trimmed vertical to the bite plane, by the required amount. It is helpful to mark this with a wax pencil on the bite plane – trimming up to, but not beyond the line. The acrylic should be trimmed back only as far as necessary to permit the tooth movement expected by the next visit. Excess trimming of acrylic may encourage the patient to posture the mandible forwards in front of the bite plane and any achieved overbite reduction will be lost. If the bite plane has not been made sufficiently high then contact with the lower incisors will quickly be eliminated as the acrylic is cut away (Figure 5.4) and to rebuild it sufficiently at the chairside is tedious. When the acrylic has been cut back sufficiently, it should be undermined to clear the palatal surfaces of the incisors and the palatal mucosa. If this is done before overbite reduction has been completed the appliance may rock when the patient occludes. The problem can be avoided by ensuring that the overbite is reduced adequately before incisor retraction commences.

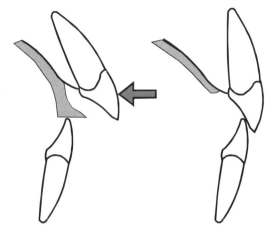

Figure 5.4 Trimming an anterior bite plane to allow overjet reduction. The fitting surface is progressively trimmed away to allow the upper incisors to be retracted while the lower incisors are still in contact with the bite plane. The leading edge of the bite plane is trimmed in a smooth curve.

Posterior bite planes

Posterior bite planes should be adjusted at the time of fitting so that there is an even contact with the posterior teeth on both sides of the arch. It is almost inevitable that some adjustment of the occlusal surface will be necessary. This should be checked with articulating paper – ensuring that the patient closes in centric – so that the occlusal surface of the bite plane is faceted to accept the opposing teeth in the centric relationship. If an anterior crossbite is being corrected the bite plane needs only to be sufficiently thick to disengage the occlusion on the anterior teeth. Quite commonly the posterior aspect of a bite plane may perforate because the acrylic is thin. Once the crossbite is corrected, the molar capping should be reduced or removed. If there is concern that the sudden removal of bite planes may allow the patient to posture the mandible to the original position then reduction may be carried out over two or three consecutive appointments.

Further reading

Cousins, A.J.P., Brown, W.A.B., Harkness, E.M. (1969) An investigation into the effect of the maxillary biteplate on the height of the lower incisor teeth. *Transactions of BSSO*, **55**: 105–109

Chapter 6

Anchorage

'Anchorage' is the term used to describe the resistance to those reactionary forces generated by the active components of the appliance. The orthodontic movement of one or more teeth is achieved by the application of a force. The reaction to this force will tend to produce movement of other teeth in the opposite direction. Anchorage control is concerned with maximizing the desired tooth movements while minimizing unwanted tooth movements. It is important to distinguish anchorage from retention (the resistance of the appliance to displacement) even though some appliance components fulfil both requirements (Figure 6.1). Clasps on upper first permanent molars,

for example, may hold the appliance in place (*retention*) while, at the same time, resisting forces of reaction to the retraction of the upper canines (*anchorage*). The two concepts must be considered separately during appliance design and adjustment as well as in the monitoring of treatment progress. Clasps sufficient for appliance retention may provide inadequate anchorage, while an appliance with excellent anchorage – for example to correct an incisor in crossbite – may be deficient in retention. Anchorage may be provided either intraorally or extraorally, but the majority of cases treated with removable appliances employ intraoral anchorage.

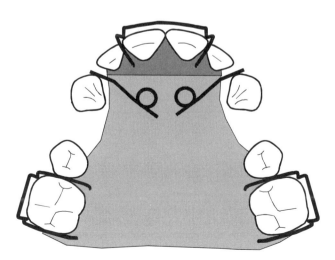

Figure 6.1 The Adams' clasps on the upper first molars and the double Adams' clasp on the central incisors provide retention and also anchorage to resist forces of retraction on the upper canines. This is an example of intramaxillary anchorage.

Intraoral anchorage

*Intra*maxillary anchorage is provided from within a single arch. This is the usual form of anchorage utilized in removable appliance treatment (Figure 6.1). *Inter*maxillary anchorage, in which one arch provides anchorage for tooth movement in the other (Figure 6.2), is commonly employed during functional and fixed appliance treatment. It cannot be used with removable appliances alone because the elastics will tend to displace the appliances. It is possible to use a removable appliance in one arch (usually the lower) to provide a point of attachment for intermaxillary elastic traction to a fixed appliance in the opposing arch. This would only be indicated when no active movement is needed in the lower arch.

Intramaxillary anchorage

This is provided mainly by the clasped teeth or those that are held in position by a short labial bow. The baseplate, however, by its close adaptation to the palate and to the teeth that are not to be moved, offers appreciable further anchorage.

In a few situations, anchorage may be described as reciprocal (Figure 6.3). This occurs when two evenly balanced groups of teeth are used to provide the anchorage for each other. An example would be the bilateral expansion of the upper arch, or closure of median diastema.

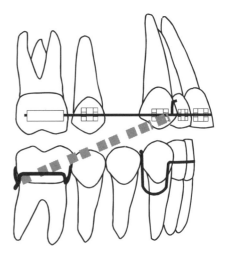

Figure 6.2 In this illustration the opposing arch is used for anchorage. Elastics are stretched between the upper fixed appliance and a lower removable appliance. For this to be effective, the retention of the lower appliance must be good. Note the modification of the molar Adams' clasp to provide a hook for the elastic. This is an example of intermaxillary anchorage.

Intermaxillary anchorage

A removable appliance can be used in conjunction with a single arch fixed appliance to provide a source of anchorage from the opposing arch. This is most common in a class II occlusion with a well-aligned lower arch. A lower removable appliance is required and hooks must be incorporated in the molar clasps

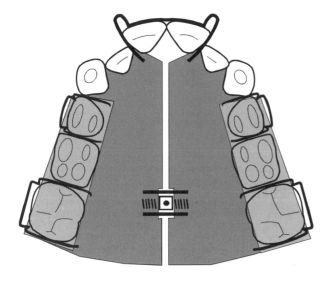

Figure 6.3 An example of reciprocal anchorage where an upper arch is being expanded. (Note that the short 'U' loop labial bow will require adjustment to permit expansion to take place.)

to provide a point of attachment for intraoral elastics, which deliver a force to the anterior aspect of the upper fixed appliance. The reciprocal force is distributed evenly to the lower arch. The method offers the advantage that a removable appliance can be fitted quickly and long before it would be possible to fit a lower fixed appliance and progress to sufficiently rigid archwires to accept class II traction.

In a class III occlusion an upper appliance can be used to deliver class III traction. Such an appliance can also be used to expand the upper arch or to procline incisors. Again, the retention must be good and hooks provided at the back of the appliance for attachment of elastics.

Anchorage consideration in appliance design

The anchorage provided by a tooth will be determined by the type of tooth movement permitted and the surface area of the root. Bodily movement, for example, offers more resistance than does tipping. With removable appliances it is not possible to prevent tipping of the anchorage teeth, but good adaptation of clasps and bows will minimize it.

When designing an appliance, it is important to incorporate as many teeth as possible into the anchorage, thus increasing the total root area of the teeth involved and consequently the resistance of the anchorage unit (Figure 6.4).

The teeth in the anchorage unit should be well clasped and there should be close contact of the acrylic to the palatal aspect of the teeth. This will help to minimize unwanted movement of the anchorage teeth.

Teeth should only be moved in small groups, except where reciprocal anchorage applies or extraoral traction is being used. As a general rule only one buccal tooth on each side should be moved at a time and canines should be moved separately from incisors. An attempt to retract the incisors together with the canines is likely to result in at least as much forward movement of the posterior anchor teeth.

Anchorage assessment

Anchorage may appear adequate when the appliance is designed but its stability needs to be assessed at each visit so that it can be reinforced

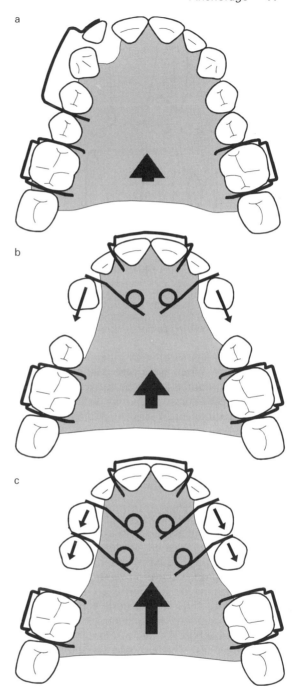

Figure 6.4 Anchorage considerations in relation to tooth movement. (a) Moving a single tooth, the other teeth in the arch and the palate provide favourable anchorage. (b) When retracting 3|3 the reaction to this movement results in forward movement of the anchorage teeth. (c) When 43|34 are retracted, there are fewer teeth available for anchorage and a greater number of teeth to be moved. The anchorage balance is less favourable.

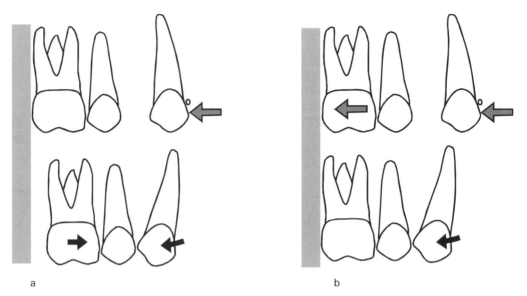

Figure 6.5 (a) When only intraoral anchorage is used, canine retraction results in forward movement of the anchor teeth. (b) Intraoral anchorage can be reinforced with extraoral thus limiting forward movement of the posterior teeth during canine retraction.

if necessary. When anchorage is solely intraoral it is very common for some movement of the anchor teeth to occur. This may be acceptable in some situations but, if space is critical, it may be wise to plan for extraoral anchorage from the start (Figure 6.5). If this is not done, it is very tempting to delay anchorage reinforcement until excessive space has been lost and must then be regained – a tedious exercise for patient and operator alike.

Assessment of anchorage stability can be difficult. Measurements taken to other teeth in the same arch are frequently misleading because all teeth contacting the baseplate may move by an equal amount leaving their relationship to each other unchanged. Reference to the opposite arch is more reliable, but here, too, teeth may move if premolars have been extracted. The most reliable base for measurement is the lower labial segment, which should be stable in the intact lower arch. If lower premolars have been extracted, however, imbricated lower incisors may start to align and the most labially placed incisor is likely to drop back. This will be shown as a slight increase in overjet and must be allowed for. Provided the baseplate contacts all the teeth that are not to be moved a change in the position of any of these teeth relative to a stable point in the lower arch gives a warning of anchorage loss. A record of the overjet, kept

while upper canines are being retracted, provides a simple and reliable way of checking anchorage stability. This measurement must be taken with the mandible in a fully retruded position on each occasion. It is easy to be misled if the patient progressively postures the mandible forwards to maintain occlusal relationships.

A sure sign that anchorage loss is occurring in the upper arch is a tendency for a buccal crossbite to develop. If the upper molars are brought forward while the transpalatal distance between them is maintained by the baseplate, they will come to oppose a narrower part of the lower arch.

Anchorage control

If anchorage loss is detected action must be taken immediately. The forces being supported by the anchorage need to be checked first. If too many teeth are being moved at the one time, or if excessive forces are being used, this must be remedied. Attention should then be paid to reinforcing the anchorage itself. The only effective way of improving anchorage is to supplement it with extraoral force. If headgear is already fitted the elastic traction may need to be strengthened. If this is already adequate then the hours of wear may need to be increased.

Extraoral anchorage

This is provided by a headgear, which can take the form of a full headcap or a high pull headgear. The direction of pull should be horizontal (occipital anchorage) or higher than this (Figure 6.6). Cervical anchorage provided by means of a neck strap cannot be used satisfactorily with a removable appliance and is not recommended unless bands have been fitted to the first molars.

Extraoral forces may be used to reinforce intraoral anchorage, but may also serve as the sole source of anchorage, for example when upper buccal segments are being retracted (Figure 6.7). When the extraoral force is the active component for tooth movement, it is referred to as extraoral traction. Extraoral force may be generated by elasticity in the headgear, by elastics connecting it to the appliance or by springs. The connection between the headgear and appliance is made by a facebow (Figure 6.8) or occasionally by 'J' hooks (Figure 6.9). It must be emphasized that these devices are potentially hazardous to the patient and to other children so the precautions discussed below must be adopted.

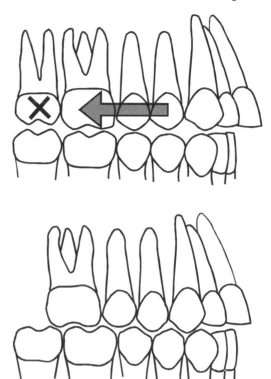

Figure 6.7 A mild class II case with minimal overjet and less than 1/2 unit class II molar relationship. In this situation, distal movement by means of headgear force to correct the molar relationship and reduce the slight overjet is often indicated. This may be associated with loss of the upper second molars.

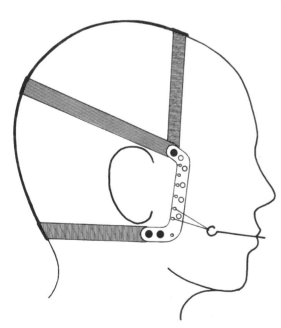

Figure 6.6 An adjustable headgear attached to a facebow by means of elastics. The direction of the force applied is slightly superior, which aids retention of the appliance.

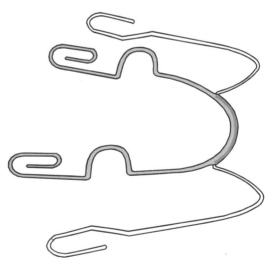

Figure 6.8 A detachable facebow. Note the recurved ends, which are designed to avoid possible injury.

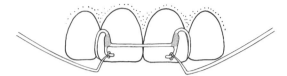

Figure 6.9 J hooks attached to hooks soldered to an anterior clasp. Note that these hooks are finished in a complete circle to avoid sharp ends.

Headgear

The options are a full headcap such as an 'Interlandi', which uses elastics to provide the force, or a high pull headgear, which may incorporate springs to generate the force. Both systems can be effective in anchorage provision. The high pull headgear is simpler and quicker to fit but is more expensive. When fitting headgear it is important to avoid a downward component of force, which tends to unseat a removable appliance. Retention may seem adequate initially but the appliance is likely to loosen with wear so that the appliance then displaces. This discourages patient cooperation and may even make the appliance unwearable. A good test of retention with headgear in place is to ask the patient to open the mouth widely and tip the

head back. If the appliance is displaced, then retention is inadequate.

When an Interlandi full headcap is used the direction of force can be varied and it is possible to attach the elastics so that the force may be directed slightly upwards as well as distally, which helps retention. The high pull headgear can only provide an upward and backward direction of pull.

It is important that the headgear should fit snugly and be comfortable. It must be kept clear of the ears. Long hair, which may make it awkward to fit a headcap, should be kept outside the straps. The straps themselves should be broad so that the load is well distributed; otherwise enthusiastic use may rub the hair away, temporarily leaving a bald spot. Some headcaps incorporate studs, which are nickel-plated and may cause an allergic reaction at the point of contact with the skin.

Facebows

Facebows may be incorporated into the baseplate if the appliance is worn only with headgear, as in the en-masse appliance (Figure 6.10). This appliance has the advantage of being the safest way of applying extraoral force. More commonly, the facebow has to be detachable

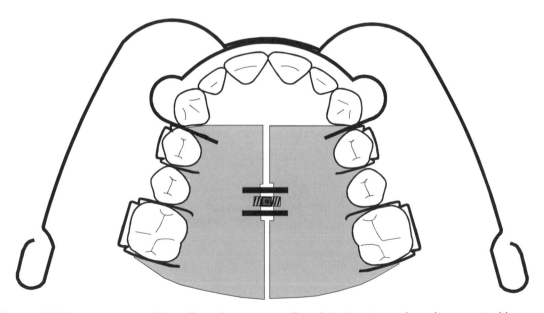

Figure 6.10 An upper removable appliance (en-masse appliance) to retract upper buccal segments with extraoral force. Adams' clasp 64|46 (0.7 mm). Mid-line screw, integral extraoral bow (1.25 mm), inner bow (1.0 mm).

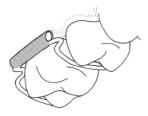

Figure 6.11 An extraoral tube soldered to an Adams' clasp.

and will be fitted into tubes (1.15 mm internal diameter) soldered to the bridges of clasps on either the molars or premolars (Figure 6.11). The tube should be soldered to the upper part of the bridge of the clasp and the ends carefully chamfered to minimize discomfort to the patient. Bending a loop in the bridge of the clasp provides an alternative method of attachment but this is less stable. The facebow must be adjusted so that it is readily inserted into the tubes and does not tend to spring out. Facebows are available commercially and come in a variety of sizes. It is best to standardize on an inner bow of 1.15 mm wire diameter to fit the tubes and with short or medium length outer arms. A selection of four inner bow lengths will fit most appliances.

It is possible to fit bands to the upper first molars to accept a facebow and fit a removable appliance over the bands. In this instance flyover clasps (Figure 6.12) must be used instead of Adams' clasps.

Fitting a facebow

The inner bow must match the arch form and length. It should lie a few millimetres labial to

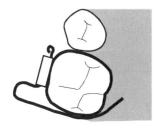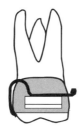

Figure 6.12 Where molar bands are fitted to first molars a flyover clasp (0.8 mm) should be used, the clasp engages the buccal tube on the molar band. This allows a removable appliance to be used in conjunction with an extraoral facebow applied to the buccal tubes on the bands.

the upper incisors (so that it does not contact them) and be at the level of the active lip line. Its length can be adjusted at the 'U' loops (see Figure 6.8). The 'U' loops may also need to be adjusted to lengthen the inner bow during treatment. The outer bow should lie just clear of the lips and cheeks with the hooks for the elastics at the level of the mesial surfaces of the first molars, about 4 cm anterior to the head cap hooks. When headgear is used with fixed appliances, the level and length of the outer arms determines the force vector applied to the teeth and thus affects their movement. With removable appliances the main concern must be that the direction of pull does not tend to unseat the appliance.

'J' hooks provide an alternative to facebows for connecting extraoral traction to an appliance (see Figure 6.9). They can be attached to spurs soldered to clasps on the upper incisors or canines. In fixed appliance treatment 'J' hooks can be valuable as a means of intruding the upper labial segment, but this is of questionable efficacy with removable appliances. To make the hooks as safe as possible it is recommended that the end be turned into a complete circle, which will still engage the hook on the appliance. The term 'O' hook is suggested.

Headgear force

For anchorage reinforcement the tension in the elastics needs to be sufficient to balance the force of reaction generated by the active components. For active retraction of buccal segments, the traction force per side should be at least 500 g. High pull headgear, which incorporates springs, can be obtained with tension gauges that are integral in the springs so that the force level can be measured. When elastic force is used, latex elastics, which are more uniform in size than commercial elastic bands, can be obtained from orthodontic supply companies. As a rule of thumb the elastic bands should be stretched to approximately twice their length. The patient should change the elastic bands every third day or before if they break.

Headgear wear

Once the initial training period with the extraoral appliance has been completed (see below) for anchorage reinforcement, it may be sufficient for the patient to wear headgear only while asleep. Where the risk of anchorage loss is not acceptable, it is wiser to start off with wear for 10–12 hours out of each 24 hours. For active retraction of buccal segments, wear for 12–14 hours out of each 24 is necessary to ensure a reasonable rate of progress. Headgear is never popular so patient motivation and monitoring are crucial to its successful use.

Safety aspects

Although trauma from 'J' hooks and facebows is very rare, it is potentially very serious. The patient is at risk if the facebow or 'J' hook becomes dislodged from the appliance. This can happen if the facebow is removed while still attached by elastics to the headcap, whether intentionally by the patient or inadvertently during play. Other children can also be at risk from contact with the external parts of headgear, facebow or 'J' hooks. A case has been reported where the facebow became displaced while the child was asleep and penetrated the eye, with subsequent loss of sight.

Facebow safety

If a detachable facebow is used then the ends that engage the tube on the molar clasp should be of the recurved design (see Figure 6.8) rather than the unprotected pointed end of the conventional design. Should the bow become detached there is less chance of facial injury. The extraoral hook should be carefully finished so that it is smooth and not prominent.

A safety strap should be fitted to prevent catapult injuries. This is a relatively rigid length of plastic, which stops the elastics being over-tensioned and helps to prevent the bow from becoming displaced inadvertently.

Safety headgear is available and is designed so that the hook attachment on the headgear (which engages the external hook of the facebow) detaches when a predetermined force level is exceeded. This reduces the risk to the patient from a catapult injury, if the facebow is pulled out of the mouth while still attached to the headcap by elastics. It does not eliminate the risk of injury if the patient dislodges the facebow while asleep and then rolls onto it.

'J' hook safety

There have been fewer cases of trauma reported with the use of 'J' hooks, but this may be due to the fact that they are not commonly used. They cannot give rise to a catapult injury. Because of their relative instability and the upward direction of traction, 'J' hooks, if they become displaced, could be potentially hazardous to the patient's eyes. The closed design of the 'O' hook avoids any sharp ends and the chances of damage must be low.

Patient instruction

When an extraoral appliance is fitted and demonstrated to a patient and parents a warning of the potential risks should also be given. This should be supported by the use of printed instructions, which should include advice to attend a hospital accident and emergency department where ophthalmic advice can be obtained should an eye injury occur.

Wear instruction and monitoring

It is usually advisable to commence with a training period and ask the patient to wear the headgear appliance in the evenings at home for the first 2 weeks after it has been fitted. The patient should then return to the surgery for the appliance to be checked. Provided it is being managed satisfactorily the patient is instructed to wear it while asleep in addition to indoor daytime wear. The headgear should be checked at every visit and the patient asked if the appliance is ever dislodged at night. The cause of this should be investigated and the headgear adjusted. If this fails to remedy the situation then the patient should not wear the headgear while asleep.

A record of the adjustment and checking of the headgear should be made in the patient's notes at every visit.

Further reading

Booth-Mason, D., Birnie, D. (1988) Penetrating eye injury from headgear. *European Journal of Orthodontics*, **10**: 111–114

Quealy, R., Usiskin, L. (1979) High pull headgear with J hooks to upper removable appliances. *British Journal of Orthodontics*, **6**: 41–42

Chapter 7

Class I malocclusions

A class I malocclusion is one in which there is no skeletal discrepancy. The relationship between the upper and lower arches is essentially normal and (barring early loss of primary molars) the molar relationship in the antero-posterior plane is class I. Within this generally satisfactory occlusal relationship there may be a number of local problems for which appliance therapy can be appropriate. The role of the removable appliance in dealing with such problems will depend upon the precise nature of the tooth displacement and whether the simple mechanics offered by removable appliances can achieve the necessary corrective movements. Two groups of cases can be identified. First, those cases where the sole problem is one of crowding and where the role of the appliance is essentially one of space maintenance. Secondly, those cases where there are local tooth displacements which can be corrected with active components (with or without associated extraction).

Many of the appliances and tooth movements described in this chapter may also be used in the treatment of both class II and class III malocclusions.

Space maintenance

In a small proportion of cases the primary problem is crowding and there are no specific local tooth displacements. Occasionally, such a malocclusion may be treated by carefully planned extractions, usually at the end of the late mixed dentition phase, without the use of any appliances (Figure 7.1).

In view of the speed with which spontaneous tooth movement can occur in children in this age range, it is often wise to maintain the arch

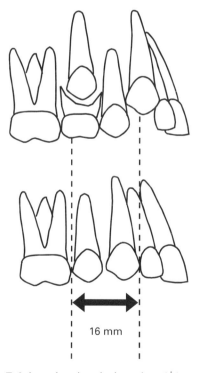

Figure 7.1 In a class I occlusion when 4|4 are extracted for the relief of buccal segment crowding, a space maintainer needs to be fitted when the space available for 53|35 reduces to 16 mm.

length while monitoring the spontaneous improvement of teeth adjacent to the extraction site. This applies particularly to maxillary canines, mandibular canines and mandibular incisors. It is often only necessary to maintain space in the upper arch because, provided the appliance does not disengage the teeth, the occlusal relationship of the molars should prevent the slower rate of spontaneous space closure in the lower arch. A suitable appliance can be simple in design because the palatal acrylic is the effective component in maintaining arch length and no active springs are required. Good retention might be provided by Adams' clasps on posterior teeth and an Adams' clasp or Southend clasp on the incisors.

Where passive space maintenance is sufficient, night-time wear will be effective. This offers a significant advantage over the fixed appliance alternatives such as the soldered or removable palatal arch attached to molar bands, which must inevitably be in place full time over an extended period.

Lower removable space maintainers can be similarly constructed but are less convenient to use than a cemented lingual arch, which may be a better choice.

Active tooth movement in Class 1 cases

- Mesio-distal tooth movement – This is commonly required to relieve crowding of canines or incisors and is a movement that is most satisfactorily carried out with removable appliances.
- Bucco-palatal movement – Buccal or palatal movement of crowded teeth is satisfactorily achieved provided that there is sufficient space in the arch.
- Posterior crossbites – Where there is a unilateral crossbite in the molar or premolar region a removable appliance can be very effective in eliminating any associated mandibular displacement on closure, while achieving the necessary maxillary expansion for correction. Such an appliance can use either a spring or a screw as an active component. The most appropriate spring in these circumstances will be the coffin spring with the appliance divided sagittally into halves. Screws may be similarly incorporated in the mid-line of an appliance. The advantage of a

screw is that it can be positioned closer to the teeth in crossbite and, by sectioning the acrylic baseplate into greater and lesser portions, the anchorage balance can be altered to give differential expansion.

Molar occlusal covering is indicated when there is a significant displacement of the mandible and is frequently used when crossbite correction is undertaken in an established dentition.

- Occlusal tooth movement – Where it is necessary to apply direct traction to a partially erupted tooth a removable appliance is the method of choice, since it takes full advantage of the vertical anchorage provided by the palatal vault through its close contact with the acrylic baseplate. In the early mixed dentition, the eruption of central and lateral incisors can be delayed as a result of an interfering factor such as a supernumerary tooth, which has to be removed surgically. More commonly, an impacted maxillary canine has to be brought into the line of the arch following surgical exposure. In either event a suitable traction point, such as a bonded hook or bracket, needs to be provided. In such cases it is usual to continue removable appliance therapy until the tooth is at approximately the same occlusal level as the naturally erupting teeth. A fixed appliance can then be used for the detailed tooth movements needed to complete treatment.
- Opening space – In the early mixed dentition it is sometimes necessary to recreate sufficient space to allow the natural eruption of an incisor which has been delayed for some reason. The principles of such treatment involve the removal of any impeding factor (such as a supernumerary tooth) and the provision of generous space into which the tooth can erupt. Since the encroaching teeth are generally tipped towards the space it is often appropriate to enlarge that space by tilting them into an upright position using springs on a removable appliance. Such treatment is often needed in the early mixed dentition, when permanent buccal teeth are not available for the placement of fixed appliances. Patients in this age range often cope better with a removable appliance than with a fixed appliance. Furthermore, any complete treatment with fixed appliances will usually have to be deferred for some

years following the successful eruption of delayed incisors. A removable appliance may provide an appropriate first treatment phase which can be followed by a period of part-time retention before definitive fixed-appliance treatment is considered.

• Space closure – Although the inflexible baseplate of a removable appliance makes general space closure difficult, if not impossible, it is occasionally helpful to move together a number of spaced incisor teeth in order to collect space nearby for erupting teeth, such as canines. Closure of a substantial mid-line diastema is rarely appropriate, as this generally requires precise control over the position of the apices of teeth if an aesthetically pleasing and stable result is to be achieved.

Short-term retention is usually all that is required following treatment of class I cases. Long-term retention is contraindicated when the prolonged use of an appliance will maintain extraction spaces in situations where natural space closure is desired after treatment.

Upper removable appliances

The following appliances may also have an application in the treatment of class II or class III occlusions and relevant comments are included where appropriate.

Tooth movements in the line of the arch

In general, single cantilever springs, boxed and guarded, are most satisfactory. The design of these springs has been discussed on p. 19. They can be used to move a tooth buccally as well as mesially or distally, but it is not generally possible to obtain appreciable palatal movement.

Incisors

Movement of incisors in the line of the arch is not commonly required but if the distance is small simple tooth movement may suffice. Closure of a median diastema may sometimes be necessary (Figure 7.2), but it should be remembered that this is a natural feature of the

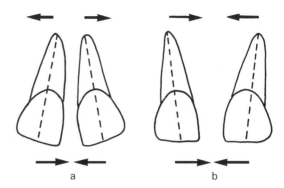

Figure 7.2 (a) A median diastema which could be closed with a removable appliance by tipping of the crowns mesially. (b) A diastema that would require a fixed appliance for space closure.

developing dentition which will often close spontaneously with the eruption of the permanent canines. A persistent median diastema may be due to a mid-line supernumerary tooth which must be removed before appliance treatment commences. Radiographs should be obtained before closure is considered.

Where upper incisors are crowded the lateral incisors may need to move distally so that alignment can proceed. If retraction of the canines has to be carried out before this the lateral incisors will often follow them, provided that the appliance does not interfere with this movement.

Incisors may need to be moved round the arch where there is a shift of centre-line, usually following asymmetric loss of a deciduous canine or first molar. Fixed appliances are usually necessary to correct significant centre-line discrepancies.

Appliance to open space for 1|1 (Figure 7.3)

Retention
Adams' clasps on 6|6.

Anchorage
The other teeth in the arch provide adequate anchorage.

Baseplate
Normal full palatal coverage.

Springs
Cantilever springs to move 2|2 distally.

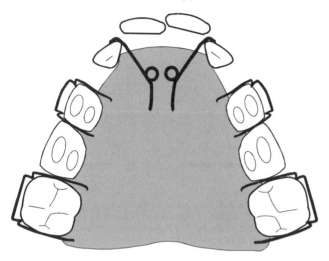

Figure 7.3 An appliance to open space for partially erupted upper central incisors for example following supernumerary removal. Clasps 6|6 (0.7 mm) and clasps on D|D (0.6 mm), palatal finger springs on 2|2.

Points to note

It is often necessary to extract the upper deciduous canines to make space, extraction of premolars may later be necessary.

Distal movement of canines

This is a very common tooth movement in class I and class II occlusions. In class II it is usually necessary to retract canines to provide space for overjet reduction and a palatal cantilever spring is the first choice. The appliance is described in Chapter 8.

In class I occlusions the main problem is one of crowding. The upper canines are usually buccally placed and a buccal canine retractor must often be used. This spring has the advantage of being able to move the canine palatally as well as distally. It can, however, easily apply excessive force with resulting unfavourable anchorage loss.

An appliance to retract canines (Figure 7.4)

Active component

Self-supported buccal canine retractors 0.5 mm spring supported in tubing with 0.5 mm internal diameter.

Baseplate

Normal full coverage.

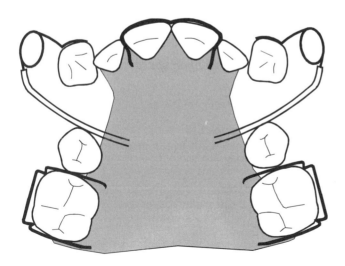

Figure 7.4 An appliance to align buccal canines. Self-supported buccal canine retractors (0.5 mm) sheathed in tubing (0.5 mm ID). Adams' clasps on 6|6. Southend clasp 1|1 (0.7 mm).

Retention
Adams' clasps on 6|6; Southend clasp on 1|1.

Anchorage
Spring pressure must be kept light.

Points to note
The buccal springs need to be adjusted carefully to avoid trauma to the cheek. Once a buccally positioned canine has been retracted sufficiently the spring can be modified to move the canine palatally.

In view of the fact that it is easy to apply excessive force with these springs a palatal cantilever spring is preferable where palatal movement is not required.

Premolars – distal movement

Where first permanent molars have been extracted and the premolars are to be retracted, a removable appliance with palatal springs is used. Usually, springs to retract first and second premolars are included in the same appliance, but they must not all be activated simultaneously or anchorage will be lost. The acrylic should be trimmed to allow the first premolars to follow the second premolars as they are retracted.

Retention of the appliance may be a problem, particularly if the second permanent molars have not erupted fully. Some retention is always required anteriorly – for example a Southend clasp on the central incisors. If the second permanent molars offer poor retention,

the first premolars may have to be clasped as well. This means that once the second premolars have been retracted sufficiently, a second appliance will be required to retract the first premolars and canines.

An appliance to retract premolars (Figure 7.5)

Active components
Palatal finger springs 54|45.

Retention
Clasps on 7|7 and 1|1 (or possibly on 4|4).

Baseplate
An anterior bite plane is indicated if the overbite is increased or if the occlusion would interfere with the premolar retraction.

Anchorage
Provided by the other teeth.

In a moderate class II case extraoral reinforcement may be necessary. When retention is poor this can present difficulties. Two appliances will be required: the first with clasps on the upper incisors and on the first premolars carrying tubes for the facebow, and the next appliance with tubes on the clasps on the second premolars.

Points to note
Sometimes there is a tendency for the second permanent molars to drift mesially in spite of the clasp. If these teeth are not fully erupted it may be helpful to incorporate palatal stops in

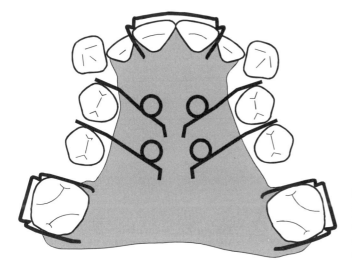

Figure 7.5 An upper removable appliance to create space for 3|3. Palatal finger springs (0.5 mm) to retract 54|45. The springs should be boxed and guarded (not shown). Adams' clasps 7|7 and double Adams' clasp 1|1 (0.7 mm).

0.5 mm hard stainless steel wire, which contact the mesial surface of the second molars, close to the gingival margin.

First permanent molars

If the first permanent molar has drifted forward following early loss of deciduous teeth, it may need to be moved back to make space for the second premolar. This is most easily done before the second permanent molar has erupted (or possibly following its extraction). It is difficult to retract both the first and second permanent molars with this type of appliance without losing anchorage, even if extraoral support is worn. Where the entire buccal segment is to be retracted, an en-masse appliance can be used (see Figure 8.15, p. 75). This will retract the premolars at the same time.

An appliance to retract a first permanent molar (Figure 7.6)

Active component
A screw with its long axis parallel to the line of the arch. This should be activated by one quarter-turn each week. (Alternatively, it is possible to use a heavy single cantilever spring in 0.7 mm wire. This should be activated by about 2 mm. The appliance is otherwise similar to that described except that the molar to be retracted is not clasped.)

Retention
Clasps on first premolars and first permanent molars.

Baseplate
An anterior bite plane is required only if there is occlusal interference with the appliance or with tooth movement.

Anchorage
This is provided by the other teeth that are contacted by the appliance and by the contact of the baseplate with the palatal vault. If only one molar is to be retracted, extraoral reinforcement may not be required. If both first permanent molars are to be retracted, then extraoral reinforcement is usually necessary. Tubes can be soldered onto the molar clasps. As the first molars move distally, the facebow should be adjusted at the 'U' loops to keep it clear of the incisors. An alternative is to use a headgear with 'J' hooks to spurs on a labial bow.

Occlusal movement

A removable appliance offers a considerable advantage in the occlusal movement of partially erupted teeth because its contact with the vault of the palate provides better anchorage for such tooth movement than does a fixed appliance. Occlusal movement is not possible unless there is a point of application to allow the spring to apply an occlusally directed force. This is simply achieved by the addition of a bonded attachment, usually to the labial surface of the tooth.

The method is particularly useful for partially erupted canines or central incisors.

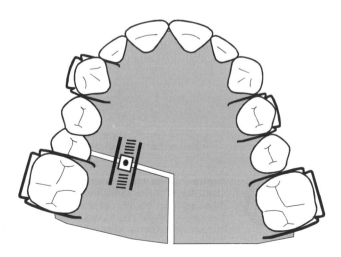

Figure 7.6 An appliance to retract 6|. Adams' clasps 63|46 (note that the screw is placed parallel to the line of the arch).

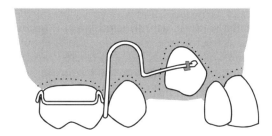

Figure 7.7 A buccal spring (0.7 mm) to move a canine occlusally. The spring engages a hook bonded onto the buccal surface of the canine.

An appliance to move a canine occlusally (Figure 7.7)

Active component
A buccal spring 0.7 mm.

Retention
Adams' clasps on 6|6.

Baseplate
As much palatal coverage as the canine position permits to offer maximum resistance to the occlusally directed force.

Anchorage
Anchorage in the vertical is provided by the acrylic in the palate.

Points to note
A point of application must be bonded to the canine (if possible to its buccal surface). This can either be a fixed appliance attachment such as a button or a short length of stainless steel wire bent into a hook. The patient must be able to engage the buccal spring onto the hook. An alternative approach is to use a latex elastic which engages the hook on the canine and is supported by a buccal arm with a fish tail which controls the direction of the elastic force.

Bucco-palatal movements

Buccal movement

A canine may erupt in a palatal position due to a slightly abnormal path of eruption or a premolar may be palatally deflected due to crowding. Before attempting to align the displaced tooth, space may have to be created. An attachment bonded to the canine will often facilitate its buccal movement while avoiding the apical component of force which may be produced by contact of a spring with the sloping cingulum. Removable appliances cannot align severely misplaced teeth. As in the case of palatally positioned incisors, stability of the tooth movement will depend to a large extent on the establishment of a good occlusal relationship with the lower arch.

A spring to move a premolar buccally (Figure 7.8)

Active component
For a premolar a 'T' spring should be used because the vertical palatal wall of the tooth can make the finger spring difficult for the

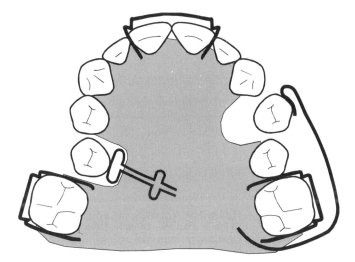

Figure 7.8 Springs to move 5| buccally and |4 palatally shown on the same appliance. A T-spring (0.5 mm) on 5|. A buccal spring (0.7 mm) on |4. Adams' clasps 6|6 and double Adams' clasp 1|1 (0.7 mm).

patient to insert. A cranked finger spring may be used for buccal movement of a canine.

Retention
Clasps on 6|6 and 1|1 or the contralateral first premolar.

Baseplate
A bite plane is usually required to clear the occlusion. Unless the overbite is reduced or the overjet reversed, an anterior bite plane is best and should be just high enough to clear the occlusion. If the overbite is reduced, thin molar capping should be used instead of an anterior bite plane.

Anchorage
This is not a problem as a large number of teeth are contacted by the baseplate and pitted against the single tooth to be moved.

Points to note
The 'T' spring should be curved so that it is clear of the palatal mucosa and should contact the tooth quite close to the cusp. If appreciable tooth movement is required, adjustment loops should be included (Figure 7.8) so that the spring may be progressively lengthened. The spring is adjusted by pulling it away from the baseplate. Excessive activation should be avoided because the spring will catch on the cusp of the tooth and make the appliance difficult to insert.

Palatal movement

Occasionally, a premolar erupts into a buccal crossbite and has to be moved palatally.

Buccally crowded canines have to be moved palatally as well as retracted and a buccal canine retractor (see Figure 7.4, p. 50) should be used. If a canine being retracted with a palatal spring has inadvertently been moved buccally, palatal movement will be required. It may be possible to modify the existing appliance by adding a buccal spring, soldered directly to the bridge of a molar clasp (Figure 7.9). If the molar clasp has to be adjusted the spring will be moved and will need its own adjustment.

A spring to move a premolar palatally (see Figure 7.8)

A self-supporting buccal arm in 0.7 mm wire entering the acrylic behind the molar clasp.

Retention
This spring does not tend to displace the appliance so retention is not a problem. Clasps on 6|6 are adequate.

Baseplate
Where occlusal interference may limit tooth movement an anterior bite plane should be included.

Anchorage
The other teeth on the same side of the arch are contacted by the baseplate and should provide adequate anchorage.

Points to note
During appliance construction the tags of clasps and springs must be kept well clear of the tooth to be moved to allow later trimming.

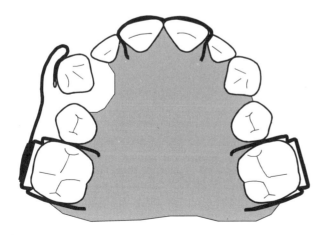

Figure 7.9 A buccally placed spring (0.7 mm) to move a canine palatally. Note the acrylic must be trimmed well clear of the palatal aspect of the tooth.

When the appliance is fitted, the baseplate must be trimmed away generously from the palatal surface of the tooth. If this is not done movements may be impeded and the gingivae may proliferate in the gap between the tooth and the baseplate. Palatal movement of a premolar or canine may be undertaken with a similar design of spring.

Bucco-palatal movement of molars

Buccal movement

Where an upper molar must be moved buccally, a 'T' spring may be successful provided that the palatal surface of the molar is reasonably vertical. The disadvantage of this spring is that it tends to displace the appliance and it may be difficult to obtain adequate retention. For this reason, a screw is sometimes preferred although it will inevitably make the appliance bulky. It is important to recognize that a molar crossbite may involve buccal displacement of the lower molar as well as palatal displacement of the upper. If this is the case then correction of the upper tooth alone will not correct the crossbite and it is usually better to use a fixed appliance to correct the positions of both teeth.

Palatal movement

It is unusual to find a single upper molar in buccal crossbite but where this does occur it should be corrected as early as possible because the tooth may over-erupt and create a functional disturbance. If the first permanent molar is affected, it should be corrected before the second molar erupts and encroaches on the space required.

Upper arch expansion

Lateral arch expansion is indicated only in well-defined circumstances. It is not a suitable procedure for the relief of crowding and if the upper incisors are crowded; space must be made by retraction of the canines. The principal indication for upper arch expansion is the existence of a unilateral crossbite associated with a lateral displacement of the mandible when the patient closes from rest to occlusion.

Such crossbites should be treated early (in the mixed dentition) to eliminate the displacement and to allow the occlusion to develop with the mandible in a centric relationship. Occlusions of this type are basically symmetrical and the apparent asymmetry is produced by the mandibular displacement, which is due to occlusal interference. Symmetrical expansion of the upper arch is required.

The presence of a unilateral crossbite with no mandibular displacement suggests a true asymmetry, either of the maxillary or the mandibular arch (or both). Examination of the arch form and the face may indicate whether this is alveolar or skeletal in origin. In either case the lack of displacement indicates that there is no underlying functional disharmony. Such an occlusion may sometimes be accepted but if treatment is to be undertaken it will be complex and is likely to involve fixed appliances.

A bilateral crossbite usually reflects an underlying dental base discrepancy, but there is rarely an associated mandibular displacement and so treatment to correct the crossbite is not mandatory. Indeed, correction of a bilateral crossbite is rarely stable and relapse is common. For these reasons, correction of a bilateral crossbite with removable appliances should not be attempted. In a few cases, the orthodontic specialist may correct a bilateral crossbite by rapid expansion to separate the mid-palatal suture. Even this treatment is prone to relapse.

An appliance for lateral expansion (Figure 7.10)

Active component
A screw (or a coffin spring) is used.

Retention
Good retention is essential. 6|6 and 4|4 should be clasped. If the latter teeth have not erupted, D|D or C|C may be clasped, but retention will be less good.

Baseplate
The baseplate is split in the mid-line to allow for the expansion. Posterior biteplanes are required for the following reasons:

- to eliminate the occlusal interference and thus the displacement
- to avoid secondary expansion of the lower arch by occlusal forces

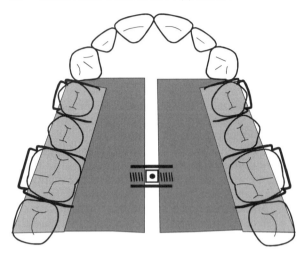

Figure 7.10 An appliance to expand the upper arch. Adams' clasps 64|46 (0.7 mm), a mid-line screw and molar capping to eliminate mandibular displacement.

- to help seat the appliance, particularly after activation.

Anchorage
The arch is to be expanded symmetrically, so anchorage is reciprocal.

Points to note
The patient should open the screw by one quarter-turn each week. If the appliance is adjusted more frequently it may not seat home fully and will become difficult to wear. The molar capping should be removed after the expansion has been completed and the appliance should continue to be worn as a retainer for at least 3 months. It is wise to cover the screw with cold-cured acrylic to prevent any unwanted movement during this stage.

Upper arch contraction

Only if there is a buccal crossbite of the upper teeth will contraction of the upper arch be necessary. This is an unusual finding associated with a broad maxillary base and a narrow mandibular base. Treatment is difficult and is best left to the orthodontic specialist. It may involve the use of an upper appliance similar to that for upper arch expansion except that the screw is opened before it is incorporated into the appliance and is closed by the patient. Simultaneous expansion of the lower arch will usually be required.

Rotations

A mildly rotated upper central incisor can be corrected with a removable appliance. Rotations of other teeth and multiple rotations can only be corrected by using a fixed appliance. Many rotations are associated with an element of apical displacement and will be difficult to correct with a removable appliance. Rotations are also particularly liable to relapse.

An appliance to derotate an upper central incisor (Figure 7.11)

Active component
A force-couple must be applied to the tooth. A labial bow and a palatal spring can generate this. If the palatal aspect of the tooth is already in the line of the arch, contact with

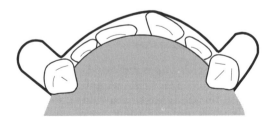

Figure 7.11 A rotated |1 to be aligned with a 'U' loop labial bow (0.7 mm). The labial bow is activated progressively. The acrylic must be cleared away from the mesial aspect of the central but maintained in contact with the disto-palatal aspect of the central incisor.

and wi
outstan

Examp
lower

Distal
where
usually
lars. Pr
out in
before
level, th
the arc
the inci
particul
canine
with a r

An app
(Figure

Active
A bucca

Retenti
Clasps
bow bu
interfer
incisors

Baseple
The bas
but thic
able app

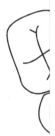

the baseplate, without a palatal spring, may be adequate.

Retention
Clasps on 6|6.

Anchorage
Little force of reaction is generated and anchorage is not a problem.

Baseplate
This is trimmed well clear of the labially displaced aspect of the tooth but should be left in contact with the palatally positioned surface.

Points to note
Space may have to be created before the rotation can be corrected. The labial bow is activated by tightening the bow at the 'U' loops. As the tooth becomes aligned, it may be necessary to incorporate a bayonet bend in the bow to keep it clear of the other incisors (see Figure 8.13, p. 73). If one aspect of the tooth is palatally positioned, a palatal spring should be used in conjunction with the labial bow.

Lower removable appliances

These have limited application and are not as well tolerated as upper removable appliances. The acrylic encroaches on the tongue-space and as the buccal undercuts on the lower permanent molars are small retention can be poor. The space available for lingual springs is limited and patients may find buccal springs uncomfortable.

Fortunately, in the majority of cases suitable for treatment by the general practitioner, the lower arch can be accepted without treatment, or with the spontaneous alignment of crowded lower teeth which can be expected to follow extractions. Where extensive lower arch treatment is required, fixed appliances are necessary.

Undercuts

There are usually undercuts on the lingual side of the lower alveolus, especially in the molar and premolar region. If the acrylic is extended into these areas during manufacture the appliance can only be removed from the work model

by breaking the plaster and can only be fitted in the mouth after considerable trimming. Since the tags of molar clasps are embedded into this area they may become loose during such trimming. Before the appliance is constructed, the undercuts should be eliminated by waxing or plastering. Alternatively, the wire tags can be shaped so that they are largely out of the undercut area which may then be trimmed away in the laboratory at the end of construction (Figure 7.12).

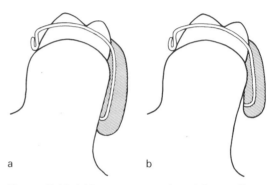

Figure 7.12 (a) Incorrect extension of the acrylic into the lingual undercut can make the appliance impossible to insert. (b) Correct finishing of the tag on the Adams' clasp allows some lingual trimming of the acrylic to facilitate fitting.

Physical limitations

The form and situation of the lower alveolus dictate that the acrylic baseplate will consist of a 'U'-shaped strip of plastic which runs parallel to the roots of the teeth. This is very different from the situation in the upper arch and trimming of the acrylic to allow movement of a tooth can easily weaken the appliance so that fracture occurs. In situations where subsequent trimming may become necessary the appliance must be selectively thickened during construction. Anchorage slip during the retraction of teeth may allow slight labial movement of the appliance, causing trauma to the lingual gingivae of the lower incisors and to the mucosa overlying the alveolus in this area. Some operators therefore prefer to replace the anterior part of the baseplate with a lingual bar, but this has the disadvantage of reducing the number of teeth and area of mucosa available for anchorage support (Figure 7.13).

started to erupt. An attempt to move both first and second permanent molars distally is likely to procline the lower incisors and, following removal of the appliance, they will drop back into muscle balance and produce secondary crowding. Occasionally, it may be necessary to remove the second permanent molar in order to move the first molar distally, but the third molar must be present and in a favourable position.

An appliance to move a lower first permanent molar distally (Figure 7.17)

Active component
A screw with a single guide pin.

Retention
Clasps on $\overline{64|46}$ or clasps on $\overline{6|6}$ and a labial bow.

Baseplate
This is split at the screw.

Anchorage
Provided by the teeth anterior to the second premolar.

Points to note
As indicated above, anchorage may be a problem but it is not practicable to provide support from outside the arch for a lower removable appliance. To minimize the forces on the anchorage, the screw should be activated by only one quarter-turn each week.

The lower removable sectional appliance

Crowding and irregularity of the lower incisors present a special problem in orthodontics. A patient may attend with a good occlusion but with irregularity of the mandibular anterior teeth, which is unacceptable. Such a patient may have had no previous orthodontic treatment or have had a course of treatment some years previously, perhaps including extractions. The problem occurs commonly in young adults and in these circumstances the sectional removable appliance described by Barrer (1975) may be useful. Lower incisors have a mean collective mesio-distal width of 22 mm (± 1.4 mm). The enamel thickness of an incisor at the contact point is 0.75 mm. The removal of 50% of the enamel from each contact point will create 3 mm of space in the incisor region. Such space may be used to effect incisor alignment provided that crowding is not too great and that any rotations are minimal.

Enamel stripping

This may be carried out before or after appliance construction, but is best done beforehand if the appliance can be supplied within a few days. Enamel removal may be carried out in several ways. Because the contact points will be tight initially it should be started with metal-backed abrasive strips. When adequate access has been gained, further enamel may be removed either in the same manner or with a

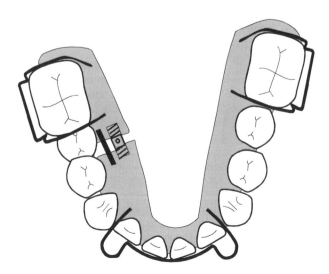

Figure 7.17 An appliance to move a $\overline{6|}$ distally. Adams' clasps on $\overline{6|6}$ (0.7 mm) and labial bow (0.7 mm). A carefully sited screw.

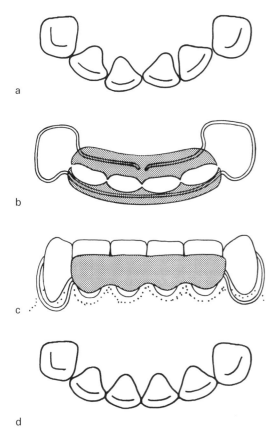

a

b

c

d

Figure 7.18 (a) Incisor crowding before interproximal stripping. (b) The sectional appliance, occlusal view. (c) The sectional appliance in position. (d) Corrected tooth position.

mechanical aid if the operator prefers. Safe sided discs, or specially designed reciprocating abraders are alternatives.

Appliance construction

The lower incisor teeth are cut off the model. If contact point reduction has not been started clinically, then plaster must be removed appropriately from the teeth at this stage. A gauge will ensure that the correct amount of tooth reduction is carried out. The teeth are set up to the anticipated new position and waxed in place. By using cold-cured acrylic to construct the appliance the need to duplicate the wax-up in plaster is avoided (Figure 7.18). A 0.7 mm stainless steel wire is laid down. This should lie in close contact with the labial surfaces of the incisors and pass around the gingival margin of

the canine without contacting the gingivae or tooth. It should then pass over the canine–premolar contact point again to follow the gingival margin of the canine without contacting it. Finally the wire should finish lingually in the mid-line.

Cold-cured acrylic (2–3 mm in thickness) is laid down over the wire buccally and lingually. It extends no further than the distal surfaces of the laterals. Dentine coloured acrylic is aesthetically most acceptable.

Clinical treatment

The appliance is inserted and adjusted to ensure suitable activation. Because the teeth have been moved during the making of the working model the appliance will probably not require activation at this stage. The patient is instructed to wear the appliance full time except for meals and sport. At subsequent appointments activation can be carried out by adjusting the distal wire loops so as to approximate further the lingual and labial acrylic bars.

Where local adjustments are necessary, appropriate trimming and the addition of small areas of cold-cured acrylic will be effective. When tooth movement is complete the passive appliance will serve as a retainer. It may be worn full time at first and then only at nights. Finally, it may be withdrawn altogether when stability seems assured. Long retention will be necessary, especially if any rotations have been corrected.

Buccal acrylic appliances

In order to overcome the dual problems of limited space for the tongue and the poor retention provided by Adams' clasps, appliances have been designed in which the acrylic rests on the buccal aspect of the lower premolars and molars. Retention is obtained by a lingually placed wire engaging the undercut on the lower first molars. A stainless steel bar is used to connect both halves of the appliance in the labial sulcus and its flexibility permits the appliance to be sprung into position. These appliances can be used to support buccal canine retracting springs or to provide molar capping when the occlusion requires disengagement.

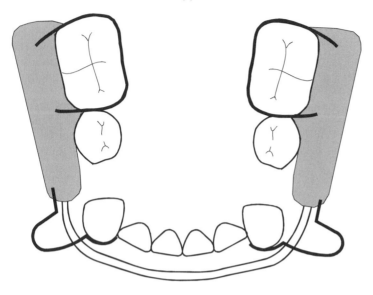

Figure 7.19 Buccal acrylic lower appliance to retract 3|3. Lingually placed Jackson clasps 6|6 (0.7 mm). Buccal stainless steel connector bar (2.0 mm × 1.0 mm half round) springs to retract the canines.

A buccal acrylic appliance to retract lower canines (Figure 7.19)

Active component
Buccal canine springs 0.7 mm.

Retention
The lingually placed Jackson clasps on the lower first molars provide retention. While undercut is often poor on the buccal surfaces of these teeth, making conventional retention difficult, the lingual undercut is often good.

Baseplate
This consists of two segments of acrylic resting on the buccal mucosa. These are connected in the mid-line by a heavy stainless steel bar, oval in cross-section, lying close to the buccal mucosa below the lower incisors.

Anchorage
This is provided by the first molars only with minimal anchorage effect from the acrylic. The original design described by Bell (1983) utilizes a lip bumper anteriorly to enhance the anchorage.

References

Barrer, H.G. (1975) Protecting the integrity of the mandibular incisor position. *Journal of Clinical Orthodontics*, **9**: 486–494

Bell, C. (1983) A modified lower removable appliance using lingual clasping and soft tissue anchorage. *British Journal of Orthodontics*, **10**: 162–163

Chapter 8

Class II malocclusions

Definition

A class II division 1 malocclusion may be defined as one in which the lower incisor edges occlude palatal to the cingulum plateau of the upper incisors. The upper incisors are either of average axial inclination or proclined. The overjet is increased and the overbite is usually increased (although it may be incomplete). The buccal segment relationship reflects the severity of the malocclusion but may be influenced by crowding or spacing in either of the arches.

Case selection

Dental base relationship

Cases that are best suited to removable appliance treatment will usually be those with a relatively mild class II dental base relationship. Occasionally the dental base relationship may be class I with the overjet being due entirely to proclination of the upper incisors. Such cases are also often well suited to treatment with removable appliances unless the incisors are clearly over-erupted.

Where the overjet is due chiefly to a class II skeletal pattern (Figure 8.1) removable appliances are inappropriate. In a growing patient, treatment with a fixed appliance or functional appliance may be better. In an adult, surgical correction may sometimes be the only satisfactory solution.

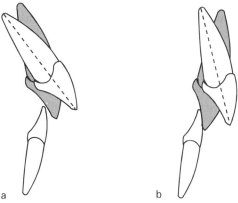

Figure 8.1 (a) A class I skeletal pattern with upper incisors proclined at the commencement of treatment, may allow satisfactory overjet reduction with a removable appliance. (b) If the overjet is reduced by means of tipping in a patient with a class II skeletal pattern with upright incisors, the appearance at the end of treatment will be unsatisfactory and a traumatic overbite may develop.

The Frankfort mandibular planes angle

This should be within normal limits. A very high angle is often associated with an anterior open bite and gross lip incompetence so such cases should be avoided. Similarly, a very low angle is often associated with excessively increased overbite together with unfavourable soft tissues – features that will not respond well to the use of removable appliances.

Soft tissues

Patients with competent, or potentially competent, lips and with a lower lip-line that is high relative to the upper incisors, may be well suited to removable appliance treatment, provided other factors are favourable. Reduction of the overjet should reposition the upper incisors so that the lower lip comes to rest labial to them and assists stability. If the patient has difficulty in achieving a lip-seal before treatment a stable result is less likely (Figure 8.2).

Occasional cases may exhibit a marked tongue thrust with an atypical swallowing behaviour – often associated with an incomplete overbite and sometimes an anterior sigmatism. The prospect for reducing the overjet in these cases is poor with any form of appliance treatment so they are best avoided.

Digit sucking habits can exaggerate a class II division 1 malocclusion. Removable appliances may be very suitable for reducing the overjet in such cases (provided the underlying skeletal pattern is not too severe) because the very presence of the appliance will frequently help the patient to overcome the habit. Parents should be warned, however, that the result might only be stable if the habit is discontinued completely.

Dental factors

Overjet

The overjet should only be modestly increased (up to about 8 mm) and should be due more to proclination of the upper incisors than to the patient's skeletal pattern. Upright incisors can only be retracted a very short distance before giving an unacceptable appearance and often an unstable result.

Lower incisors

One of the aims of treatment for a class II division 1 case is that the average labio-lingual position of the lower incisors should be accepted. (The relief of crowding will allow some spontaneous alignment of individual labially or lingually crowded incisors.) In a small number of cases the lower incisors are also proclined, producing a consequent bi-maxillary

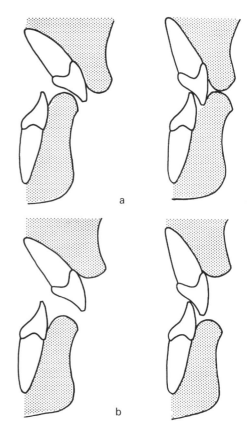

Figure 8.2 (a) Favourable soft tissue pattern for overjet reduction in a class II division 1 case. (b) Unfavourable soft tissue pattern at the end of treatment, the lower lip does not cover the upper incisor tips.

proclination. Reduction of the overjet in these cases will usually demand lingual movement of the lower incisor crowns, which will entail fixed appliances. Conversely, the lower incisors are, on occasion, excessively retroclined and these cases also require fixed appliances to achieve a satisfactory inter-incisor angulation.

Overbite

In a growing patient, a moderate increase of overbite can be reduced by the use of a removable appliance incorporating an anterior bite plate. An overbite that is excessive and perhaps causing trauma to the palatal gingivae may be less amenable to removable appliance treatment, particularly if it is associated with a low Frankfort mandibular planes angle. If the overbite is incomplete, due to adaptive tongue behaviour or to a habit, then a satisfactory correction is usually achieved following reduction of the overjet. Where an anterior open bite exists, associated with skeletal factors or with unfavourable tongue behaviour, it may not be possible to achieve a satisfactory incisal relationship.

Crowding

The degree of crowding should be such that alignment can be achieved by simple movements. Gross displacement of individual teeth, marked rotations, apical malpositions or distal inclination of the canines are contraindications to removable appliance treatment.

Most removable appliance treatments only involve active tooth movement in the upper arch. The lower arch must therefore either be acceptable or else be one in which alignment will occur naturally as the result of relief of crowding produced by the extraction of lower first premolars. Such movements occur best in a growing child and once the pubertal growth spurt is past there is a marked reduction in the amount of natural alignment that will take place. This is especially relevant for female patients in whom growth ceases earlier (Stephens, 1983).

Missing teeth and those of doubtful prognosis

Where teeth are congenitally absent it is often impossible to establish a satisfactory contact point by the use of removable appliances alone. Missing lower second premolars, for example, will almost invariably require fixed appliances to achieve satisfactory contact points. Similarly, where teeth are of a doubtful prognosis, especially first molars, satisfactory results are difficult to achieve with removable appliances alone. Occasionally, sensibly planned extractions, carried out at an early stage, may allow satisfactory contacts to develop.

Aims of treatment

The aims of treatment for a class II division 1 malocclusion are the reduction of the overbite

and overjet, the relief of crowding, an improvement in appearance and the achievement of a stable result.

Overjet reduction must be carried out solely by alteration of the angulation of the upper incisors, the labio-lingual position of the lower incisors has to be accepted because it cannot be reliably altered by removable appliances. The stability of the result will depend upon the upper incisors being retracted to a position where they are under the control of the lower lip. If this cannot be achieved then the lower lip may cause the upper incisors to relapse.

In adult patients, treatment may be undertaken with the understanding that retention must be on a permanent basis because a stable result cannot be achieved. This is not an option to be undertaken lightly and the patient must understand, before treatment commences, that permanent retention will be necessary.

Extraction choice

Removable appliances offer two main avenues for the management of a class II division 1 malocclusion. The more common approach involves the extraction of upper first premolars (and sometimes also the lower first premolars) to relieve crowding while providing space for canine retraction and overjet reduction. A much smaller group of patients can (provided they are still growing) be treated without premolar extractions, using headgear to move the upper buccal segments distally prior to reduction of the overjet.

The decision concerning extraction depends upon a careful assessment of the malocclusion and will be decided by the severity of the malocclusion (as demonstrated by the molar relationship and the overjet) as well as on the degree of crowding. Some suggested guidelines are given below.

Molar relationship class I or less than half unit class II

In all cases, the degree of crowding in the lower arch provides a guide to lower arch extraction. With less than half a unit class II molar relationship and an uncrowded lower arch, lower premolar extractions are contraindicated and the upper arch can usually be treated by distal

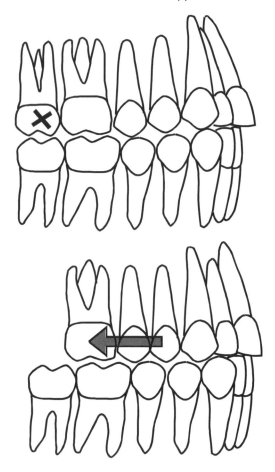

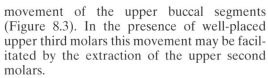

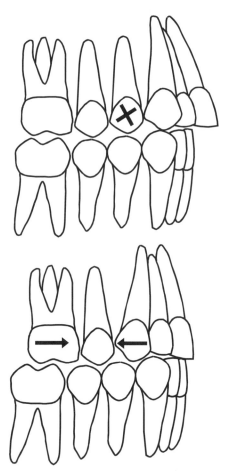

Figure 8.3 A class II division 1 occlusion with a well aligned lower arch and a molar relationship of half a unit class II or less. Premolar extractions in this type of occlusion would give too much space. Extraction of upper second molars, the use of extraoral traction to move back the buccal segments and reduce the overjet, is more appropriate treatment.

Figure 8.4 Molar relationship more than half unit class II, but a well aligned lower arch. In such cases it is sometimes possible to extract the upper first premolars only, finishing with a class II molar relationship.

movement of the upper buccal segments (Figure 8.3). In the presence of well-placed upper third molars this movement may be facilitated by the extraction of the upper second molars.

If the lower arch is mildly crowded the extraction of all four first premolars may be indicated, depending upon the age and sex of the patient. If the second molars have erupted fully and the occlusion is well established, then extraction of the lower first premolars may leave residual space. In such cases, the extraction of lower second premolars may well be the better choice but will necessitate the use of fixed appliances.

Molar relationship more than half a unit class II

Where there is an uncrowded lower arch it may be possible to extract the upper first premolars, retract the canines and reduce the overjet. This will allow the first molars to establish a class II buccal segment relationship, which will be acceptable because units have only been lost from the upper arch (Figure 8.4). In the treatment of such a case, extraoral anchorage may be needed to prevent excessive forward movement of the upper first molars during treatment.

If the lower arch is mildly crowded and the patient is of an appropriate age, the extraction

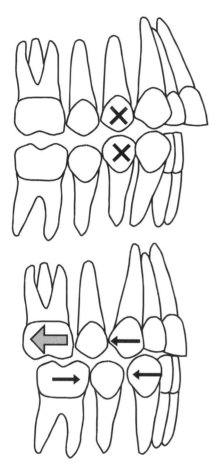

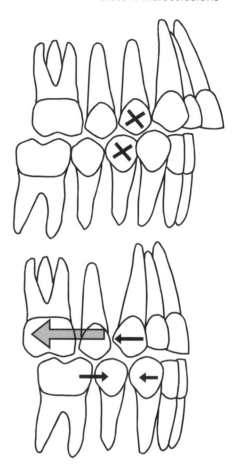

Figure 8.5 Molar relationship more than half unit class II with a crowded lower arch. Provided the lower arch can be expected to improve spontaneously, the extraction of all four first premolars and the use of upper removable appliances can treat this occlusion. Extraoral support may well be needed in such cases.

Figure 8.6 Molar relationship a full unit class II molar with a crowded lower arch may be treated with removable appliances provided that the underlying skeletal pattern is moderate. Extraoral support will be required.

of all four first premolars can be considered, allowing for spontaneous alignment of the lower arch and the use of appliances in the upper arch. Reinforcement of the anchorage by the use of extraoral forces may be necessary in such cases to hold the upper molars in place as the buccal occlusion corrects (Figure 8.5).

Molar relationship fully class II

Caution – many patients with an uncrowded lower arch and a full class II molar relationship also have a marked skeletal II dental base relationship. These should be avoided because the overjet cannot be satisfactorily reduced by tipping the incisors. Cases suitable for removable appliance treatment are likely to have mild upper arch crowding and only a slightly increased overjet.

If there is mild lower arch crowding and the patient is of an appropriate age then the extraction of all four first premolars might be considered with the wear of headgear to move the upper molars distally into a class I relationship, but only if the patient does not have a marked skeletal II base (Figure 8.6).

The presence of severe lower arch crowding with a class II molar relationship indicates an extremely difficult case which will require treatment by a specialist.

Treatment methods

As has already been stated, the two main avenues of treatment are likely to involve either premolar extractions or second molar extractions. Premolar extraction cases constitute by far the larger group and will be described first.

Premolar extraction cases

The upper canines require retraction into a class I relationship with the lowers when the latter are in an uncrowded position. Any necessary overbite reduction can be achieved at the same time with an anterior bite plane. A second appliance is then required to reduce the overjet, while maintaining overbite reduction with an anterior bite plane and holding the canines in their new position.

Appliance design

Appliances are required for the three distinct stages and will be described below.

1. Canine retraction and overbite reduction

The ideal spring for canine retraction is the palatal finger spring, boxed and guarded. This

is best made in 0.5 mm stainless steel wire. First molar clasps are required for retention, together with a clasp on the incisors. Overbite reduction is produced by a flat anterior bite plate, which is just sufficiently deep to contact the lower incisors evenly (Figure 8.7). Where extraoral support is required, tubes should be added to the molar clasps to accept the facebow.

Where an upper canine is crowded buccally a standard palatal finger spring is unsuitable. In such cases a supported buccal canine retractor in 0.5 mm wire is recommended – although this is, in many ways, less satisfactory. Overbite reduction and extraoral support may be achieved as described above.

2. Overjet reduction

Once the canines have been retracted into class I with the lowers and the overbite has been reduced, overjet reduction can commence, using a Roberts' retractor. The appliance should incorporate stops mesial to the canines (to prevent their forward relapse) and an anterior bite plate sufficiently thick to maintain the existing overbite reduction. In order to permit overjet reduction the acrylic must be hollowed out on the palatal aspect of the fitting surface. This should be carried out progressively during overjet reduction (Figure 8.8). Towards the end of this process the canine stops can be removed

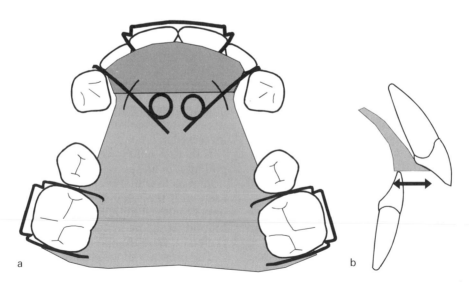

Figure 8.7 (a) An appliance with palatal canine retractors (0.5 mm) and a double Adams' clasp on 1|1 (0.7 mm). (b) The upper bite plane should only extend sufficiently posteriorly just to engage the lower incisors.

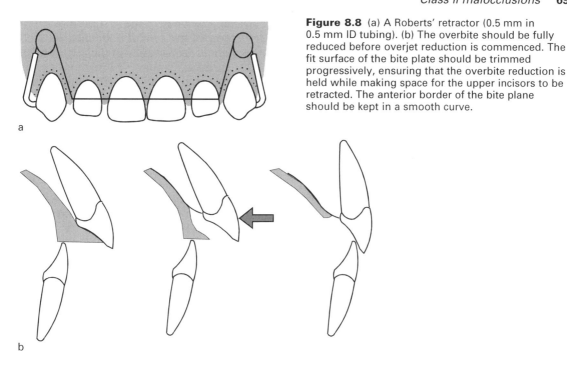

a

b

Figure 8.8 (a) A Roberts' retractor (0.5 mm in 0.5 mm ID tubing). (b) The overbite should be fully reduced before overjet reduction is commenced. The fit surface of the bite plate should be trimmed progressively, ensuring that the overbite reduction is held while making space for the upper incisors to be retracted. The anterior border of the bite plane should be kept in a smooth curve.

as the upper incisors are retracted into contact with the lower. Extraoral support will sometimes still be necessary during this phase of treatment.

In a few mild cases it is possible to correct the canines and the incisors with a single appliance. The design might include palatal canine springs and a reverse loop labial bow (Figure 8.9). Care must be taken to activate only the palatal springs until the canines are sufficiently retracted. At that stage these springs can be made passive and the reverse loop labial bow can be activated. Because these bows are extremely inflexible, many operators prefer to divide the bow at the mid-line to make it more flexible to carry out overjet reduction.

This approach is only indicated where there is a very small overjet or where mild crowding of the incisors exists and a reverse labial bow is suitable for alignment.

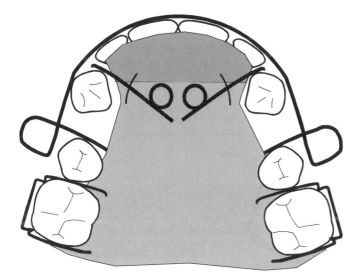

Figure 8.9 A single appliance used for canine retraction and reduction of a small overjet. Canine spring (0.5 mm), reverse loop labial bow (0.7 mm). The canine retraction must be completed first and it is sometimes advantageous to cold cure the canine springs in a passive position once the canines have been retracted. The reverse loop labial bow may then be activated to reduce the overjet.

3. Retention

The reduced overjet requires retention which is best provided by a purpose-made retainer with cribs on upper first molars and a 'U' loop labial bow. The Roberts' retractor is not ideal for retention because it is too flexible and can, over a period of time, become distorted. When a reverse loop labial bow is being used for overjet reduction, this may be used for a retention phase.

Extraoral anchorage

If the molars are not class I at the outset of a four premolar extraction case extraoral support must be considered. The use of extraoral force supports the molars during canine retraction and aids the achievement of a class I molar relationship. Sometimes it will only be needed during canine retraction; sometimes through the entire treatment. The choice will depend upon the severity of the problem and clinical judgement must be used in the management of each case.

Where first premolars are extracted from the upper arch alone there should be a class II molar relationship at the end of the treatment. Extraoral support will be required only if the molar relationship was originally a half-unit class II or more.

Canine retraction

Before the overjet can be reduced and the incisors aligned the upper canines must be retracted. Space can be provided for this either by extraction (usually of the first premolars) or by retraction of the buccal segments. Removable appliances are suitable for the retraction of mesially inclined canines. Retraction of the incisors must be delayed until the canines have been corrected or else anchorage will be overloaded. For a canine in the line of the arch a palatal spring is best, but a buccal spring is better for a buccally crowded tooth.

Provided that the lower incisors and canines are well aligned the upper canines should be retracted into a class I relationship with the lowers. If the canines are to be retracted by more than half a tooth-width then extraoral support must be considered. Where a class II skeletal pattern precludes the establishment of a normal incisor relationship (i.e. if a residual overjet is to be accepted or if the upper incisors will be retroclined after retraction) the canines may not have to be moved so far. If slight lower incisor crowding is to be accepted, the upper canines need to be retracted further unless a residual overjet or upper incisor crowding is to be accepted.

An appliance to retract upper canines (Figure 8 .10)

Active components
Where the canines are in the line of the arch, palatal cantilever springs, boxed and guarded, should be used. Where a canine must be moved palatally as well as distally a palatal spring is not suitable and a buccal spring is necessary in order to engage the tooth correctly and to

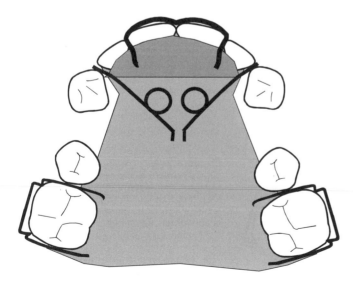

Figure 8.10 An appliance to retract upper canines. Palatal cantilever springs (0.5 mm) boxed and guarded. Southend clasp (0.7 mm). Adams' clasp (0.7 mm). A flat anterior bite plane.

deliver a palatal component of force (see Figure 3.6, p. 18). This can be a retractor, made from 0.5 mm wire supported in tubing, or a self-supporting spring made from 0.7 mm wire.

Retention

Clasps will be needed on first permanent molars. A double Adams' clasp or a Southend clasp may be used on the central incisors. This is most important if anchorage is to be supplemented by extraoral traction.

Anchorage

Retraction of canines places demands on anchorage. It is difficult to avoid some anchorage loss without the use of headgear. Unless there is space to spare, extraoral support will probably be necessary either with a facebow to tubes on the molar clasps, or with 'J' hooks to the anterior part of the appliance.

Baseplate

Usually an anterior bite plane will be required in class II division 1 cases to reduce the overbite and occasionally to clear the occlusion.

Points to note

The spring should not be activated until the tooth is close to the occlusal level otherwise its eruption will be impeded. The point of contact of the spring with the tooth is important and, particularly with palatal springs, unwanted buccal movement should be watched for. Some orthodontists incorporate a labial bow (see Figure 3.25, p. 27) into this appliance to prevent buccal drift of the canines but it is better to ensure that the springs are correctly made and adjusted. Palatal springs should be activated by just less than half a canine tooth width (3 mm).

Care must be taken not to overactivate buccal springs because they are capable of generating large forces which may overload the anchorage, causing loss of space and an increase in overjet. Self-supporting buccal springs should only be activated by about 1 mm. Supported buccal springs may be activated by 2 mm.

Incisor retraction

In class II, division 1 cases, overjet reduction is one of the main treatment objectives. Space must first be created by retraction of the upper canines. If the incisors are irregular or the overjet is small (less than 4 mm), alignment may be carried out on the same appliance as canine retraction (see Figure 3.25, p. 27) by the incorporation of a labial bow. After canine retraction, the bow is modified (see Figure 3.23, p. 25) to retract the incisors. Overbite reduction is undertaken during canine retraction but the biteplate continues in use during overjet reduction to maintain the lower incisor depression (and to reduce the overbite further, should this be necessary).

Where the overjet is large (more than 4 mm) it is preferable to use a second appliance to reduce it with a light flexible bow such as Roberts' retractor (Figure 8.11). This has a range of action sufficient to permit continuous

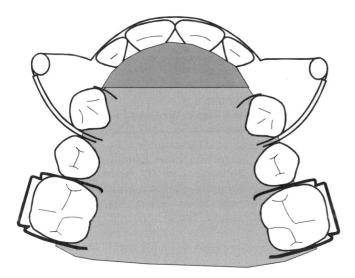

Figure 8.11 An appliance to retract the upper incisors. A Roberts' retractor (0.5 mm) sheathed in tubing (0.5 mm ID). Stops on 3|3. Cribs on 6|6 (0.6 mm). A bite plane to maintain overbite reduction.

tooth movement with adjustments at 4–6 weekly intervals. (Whether one or two appliances are used, the canines must be retracted fully before the palatal acrylic is trimmed and the labial bow activated.)

Stability of overbite reduction depends on the establishment of a stable contact between upper and lower incisors. If the interincisal angle (angulation between the long axes of the upper and lower incisors) is appreciably greater than 140 degrees, the overbite will deepen when appliances are discontinued. Only mild class II, division 1 cases should be treated with removable appliances. If the skeletal pattern is markedly class II, if the overjet is very large, or if the incisors are not proclined, there is little chance of obtaining good results with removable appliances. These patients will require a more complex treatment.

An appliance to retract the upper incisors (Figure 8.11)

Active component
A Roberts' retractor.

Retention
Clasps on 6|6.

Anchorage
This is provided principally by the first permanent molars. If space is very short, anchorage may be reinforced by extraoral traction applied via tubes on the molar clasps.

Baseplate
A bite plane is required to maintain or produce overbite reduction. The depth of the bite plane will depend upon the size of overjet. If the overbite has already been reduced, the bite plane should be made almost level with the lateral incisor edges. Bite plane adjustment is described on p. 38. Soft stainless steel wire stops are included to prevent relapse of the canine retraction.

Points to note
Anchorage demands during incisor retraction are generally less than those during canine retraction. Occasionally, problems may be encountered where there is a strong contraction of the lower lip behind the upper incisors but a full bite plane to the height of the incisors will usually prevent this. Where there is a

danger of anchorage loss, tubes should be soldered to the first molar clasps and the anchorage reinforced with headgear. Alternative springs for retraction of the incisors are a high labial arch with apron spring, a split labial bow, self-straightening wires or the extended bow as described in Chapter 3.

Retraction of individual incisors

Occasionally, individual incisors have to be retracted. An incisor, which is more labially placed than the others, will show a tendency to relapse. To allow for this, the tooth should, if possible, be over-corrected. Precise control over individual tooth position is more readily obtained with a less flexible bow than may be used for the reduction of a large overjet (Figure 8.12).

An appliance to retract a prominent upper central incisor

Active component
A labial bow in 0.7 mm wire, either with reverse loops (see Figure 3.25, p. 27) or 'U' loops (see Figure 3.21, p. 25) is recommended. An extended bow can also be used (see Figure 3.27, p. 27).

Retention
Clasps on 6|6.

Anchorage
Adequate anchorage is provided by the first molars.

Baseplate
An anterior bite plane should be used to ensure overbite reduction and to allow full retraction of the incisors.

Points to note
Space will, again, need to be provided by the retraction of the canines. This may be carried out using palatal springs on the same appliance. Over-correction of a labially placed incisor, while desirable, can only be carried out when the lower incisors permit. Upper incisor irregularity may often reflect that of the lower incisors and permanent correction of the upper incisor positions may not be possible unless the lowers are also to be aligned. The bow should be adjusted later with bayonet bends (Figure

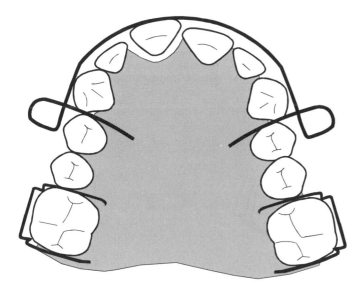

Figure 8.12 An appliance to retract a prominent upper central incisor.

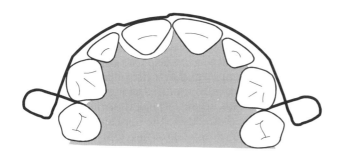

Figure 8.13 Once the retraction has commenced, it may be necessary to add bayonet bends mesial and distal to the central incisor to ensure that the force of the 'U' loop labial bow is applied to the incisor.

8.13) on either side of the prominent tooth. This ensures that the bow acts only on the prominent incisor. Subsequently the bow may be activated at the 'U' loops.

Treatment in second molar extraction cases

Distal movement

Where the lower arch is uncrowded, or exhibits only very mild crowding, the buccal segment relationships may best be corrected by the use of extraoral force to move the upper buccal segments distally. It is not practical, however, to move the buccal segments more than half a unit in this manner. The movement of the upper buccal segments can be facilitated by the extraction of upper second molars (providing the upper third molars are present and well placed).

Appliance design

A variety of appliance designs may be used. All of them must make provision for the intermolar width to be increased during distal movement to compensate for the shape of the arch and to prevent a crossbite from developing. An appliance may either incorporate screws or springs with headgear support, or else rely solely on extraoral force to achieve the movement (an 'en-masse' appliance). The third method, using fixed appliance techniques, is to cement molar bands and apply the extraoral force directly to these.

An appliance to retract upper first molars: twin screw appliance (Figure 8.14)

Active components

This appliance incorporates two screws, placed at a slight angle to allow for upper arch width

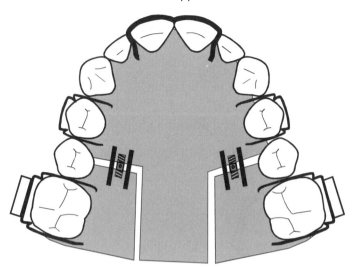

Figure 8.14 The twin-screw appliance. This appliance is particularly useful when different amounts of movement are required on each side. Molar headgear tubes are soldered to the Adams' clasps (1.15 mm ID).

correction. Soldered tubes will be required on the first molar clasps to take an extraoral face-bow.

Retention
Clasps are required on first molars and possibly also on first premolars.

Anchorage
Anchorage is provided by the contact of the baseplate with the other teeth in the arch and supported by extraoral anchorage.

Baseplate
The baseplate is split in the premolar region. The acrylic may be trimmed well clear of the second premolars, or alternatively it may be left in contact to allow the second premolars to be moved back simultaneously as the screw is activated

Points to note
A disadvantage of this method is that if the headgear is not worn but the screw continues to be turned the reaction will produce a rapid increase in the overjet.

After the molars have been successfully corrected to a class I relationship, further appliances will be required to retract the first premolars and canines and then to reduce the overjet, using similar appliances to those described for premolar extraction cases. Extraoral support will invariably still be required.

An appliance to move buccal segments distally: the 'en-masse' appliance (Figure 8.15)

This appliance derives its effect solely from extraoral force. Clasps are usually fitted on the first molars and first premolars with expansion being achieved either with a coffin spring or a mid-line screw. The extraoral force can be applied directly to the appliance by incorporating an integral facebow into the acrylic. The appliance is inactive without the headgear so there is no risk of producing an increase in overjet. Headgear needs to be worn for a minimum of 14 hours each day to achieve satisfactory distal movement. If this is successful, it is common to find reduction of the overjet taking place at the same time. The distal movement can be facilitated by the extraction of the upper second molars in those cases where third molars are present and of a good size. A second appliance to retract the canines and reduce the overjet will usually be required.

Active components
The elastic of the headgear and a mid-line screw or coffin spring to provide expansion.

Retention
Clasps on the first premolars and first molars.

Anchorage
The anchorage is derived solely from the elastic or spring tension of the headgear. The facebow is normally integral to the appliance.

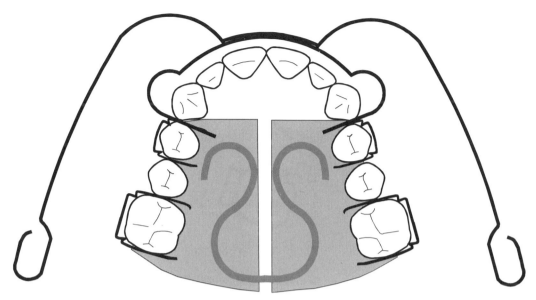

Figure 8.15 An appliance to move upper buccal segments distally. The extraoral bow is embedded into the acrylic of the appliance. A coffin spring (1.25 mm) is available for expansion.

Baseplate

This is normally trimmed away from behind the upper incisors, but is split in the mid-line to permit compensating expansion.

Points to note

To achieve satisfactory buccal segment movement the headgear needs to be worn for a minimum of 14 hours each day – a longer period than would be needed to support a screw-plate. Some overjet reduction may occur at the same time.

The mid-line screw should be adjusted by the operator so that the buccal segments diverge as they move distally, preserving the transverse arch relationship and avoiding the creation of a crossbite. One quarter turn every 4–6 weeks is usually adequate. Alternatively, if a coffin spring is used, this will require expansion by the operator at the routine visits. The correction of an existing crossbite requires more expansion so a mid-line screw should be used and can be adjusted weekly by the patient.

Because the facebow is integral with the appliance, this is one of the safest ways of applying extraoral force to the upper arch.

Bands on first molars

Bands may be placed on upper first molars with buccal tubes which accept the inner arms of the facebow directly, enabling the molars to be moved distally with extraoral force. The inner arch of the facebow should be expanded slightly to provide arch-width correction and the outer arms should be directed upwards and backwards and attached to a safety headgear. The molars may become slightly mobile and care should be taken that they are not extruded by a downward component force from the facebow.

It is common to find that the premolars follow the molars distally due to the effect of the transeptal fibres. If this does not occur a removable appliance can be fitted over the molar bands once these teeth are in a class I relationship so that premolars and/or canines can be retracted with palatal finger springs. A final appliance can also be clipped over the molar bands so that extraoral support can, if necessary, be continued during overjet reduction.

An appliance to facilitate distal movement of upper molars with bands and extraoral traction (Figure 8.16)

Active components

Palatal springs in 6 mm wire can engage both upper first molars to support the distal force applied by the facebow directly to the molar bands.

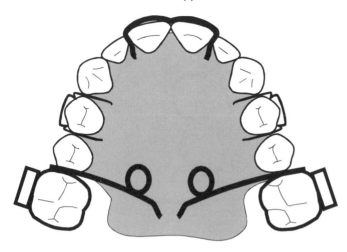

Figure 8.16 An appliance to use with molar bands. The headgear is applied directly to the tubes on the bands. The unsupported springs (0.6 mm) should only be activated by 1–2 mm.

Points to note

The removable appliance is worn full time and enhances the effect of the headgear, which is being applied directly to the molar bands. It is particularly useful when unilateral distal movement of a molar is required. In such a case only a unilateral spring is necessary with the molar on the opposite side being clasped with a flyover clasp.

Class II division 2 malocclusion

Only a small proportion of such cases are amenable to removable appliance treatment. Where the overbite is increased and potentially traumatic, fixed appliances will be usually necessary to establish a satisfactory interincisor angle. If, however, the overbite is increased but not potentially traumatic and the upper arch crowding is relatively mild with a good lower arch then a class II division 2 malocclusion can be treated utilizing a distal movement technique.

Cases where there is sufficient crowding to warrant premolar extractions, either in both arches or the upper arch alone are not suitable for removable appliance treatment. Extraoral support will be necessary to achieve distal movement of the buccal segments to a class I relationship but normally a full-time removable appliance will be indicated as overbite reduction is likely to be necessary and it is difficult to achieve this with partial wear. Once the molar relationship is corrected to a class I then retraction of canines

and alignment of the lateral incisors can be carried out. A 'U' loop labial bow may be appropriate to align the lateral incisors – but only if a limited amount of control of rotation can be achieved. In a growing patient, some improvement in the interincisor angulation may be found as a result of some proclination of the upper incisors during the overbite reduction stage.

The upper lateral incisors have an inherent tendency to relapse and will require pericision and long-term retention following alignment.

References

Stephens, C.D. (1983) Factors affecting the rate of spontaneous space closure at the site of extracted mandibular first premolars. *British Journal of Orthodontics*, **10**: 93–97

Further reading

Battagel, J.M., Ryan, A. (1998) Treatment changes in class I and mild class II malocclusions using the *en-masse* appliance. *European Journal of Orthodontics*, **20**: 5–15

Cetlin, N.M., ten Hove, A. (1983) Non extraction treatment. *Journal of Clinical Orthodontics*, **17**: 396–413

Orton, H.S., Battagel, J.M., Ferguson, R., Ferman, A.M. (1996) Distal movement of buccal segments with the *en-masse* appliance. *American Journal of Orthodontics*, **109**: 379–385

Stephens, C.D., Lloyd, T.G. (1980) Changes in molar occlusion after extraction of all first pre-molars, a follow up study of class II division 1 cases treated with removable appliances. *British Journal of Orthodontics*, **7**: 139–144

Chapter 9

Class III malocclusions

A class III malocclusion is one in which there is a reversed overjet on at least one incisor. This is frequently associated with a displacing activity of the mandible where an initial contact causes a forward displacement into the reversed overjet.

Case selection

Removable appliances are only suitable for treating the more mild class III cases. They are, however, particularly useful for interceptive treatment in the mixed dentition stage.

There are a number of factors to consider in the selection of cases, which are suitable for treatment with removable appliances.

Favourable factors

Skeletal pattern

The underlying skeletal pattern is relevant in the identification of those patients with reversed overjets who are suitable for treatment with removable appliances. The skeletal pattern should be class I or only mildly class III (although it should be remembered that a displacing activity of the mandible would make the class III skeletal pattern appear more severe). The Frankfort mandibular planes angle should be average or reduced.

Overjet and overbite

The reversed overjet should be small and coupled with a forward displacement of the

mandible (Figure 9.1). An increased overbite will favour the correction of a reversed overjet because there will still be a positive overbite after treatment. Cases which have only one or two central incisors in lingual occlusion and which involve a displacing activity are usually well suited to removable appliance treatment.

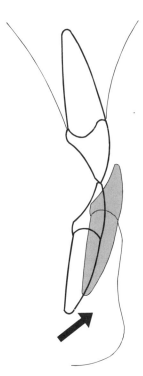

Figure 9.1 Forward displacement of the mandible which results in a class III incisor relationship. This can usually be treated with a removable appliance.

Even a reversed overjet on four incisors may be treatable if there is a displacing activity.

Incisor angulation

The upper incisors should, ideally, be slightly retroclined or of average axial inclination. Retroclined upper incisors are suited to proclination with removable appliances. The lower labial segment should have an average axial inclination or be slightly proclined.

Buccal crossbite

A unilateral crossbite often accompanies a mild class III occlusion. If there is an associated displacement of the mandible to one side, the patient should be examined with the mandible in the non-displaced position. A unilateral crossbite associated with a mild skeletal class III pattern and with only one incisor in crossbite, may still be favourable for correction.

Lower arch considerations

Ideally, the lower arch should be well aligned – this is a common feature of class III occlusions and relates to the size of the mandible. In some cases, where the reverse overjet is largely a feature of crowding, lower canine and incisor crowding may be sufficient to justify first premolar extractions. Spontaneous alignment of the crowded lower incisors will occur in the growing patient. This is aided by the fitting of an upper removable appliance with molar capping which will help to eliminate the displacement and allow crowded and labially placed incisors to align lingually.

Age factors

One of the commonest interceptive treatments in the early mixed dentition is the correction of a reverse overjet on recently erupted central incisors.

An upper central incisor may erupt in lingual occlusion because it has been deflected palatally by delayed shedding of its predecessor, or because of a slightly abnormal path of eruption. If the palatal deflection is recognized before the tooth has reached the occlusal level, it may be possible to correct it simply by extracting the retained deciduous tooth and instructing the patient to bite on a tongue spat-

ula. Once an overbite has been established this measure is not usually successful and an appliance will be required. Provided there is a displacing activity, it is sensible to consider early appliance treatment to avoid traumatic occlusion with the lower incisors. This may be associated with gingival recession and unsightly attrition to the labial faces of the upper incisors. Early treatment also reduces the chance that later erupting teeth may develop in lingual occlusion.

When early treatment is to be carried out, the parents should be informed that this is an interceptive phase of treatment which aims to deal with local problems and that further treatment may be required when the permanent dentition is established.

Upper lateral incisors, which erupt palatally, are a sign of crowding. If this is detected early, extraction of the deciduous canines, while the lateral incisors are erupting may allow spontaneous correction. Usually, however, the lateral incisors will need to be proclined with an appliance. Such movement should be undertaken when the unerupted canines are still high and before they have moved down labial to the roots of the lateral incisors. If this has already happened, correction of the lateral incisors must be delayed until such time as it is possible to retract the canines.

Correction of a reverse overjet can be considered in the later stages of the mixed dentition but, as the permanent dentition becomes established there is an increasing chance of an underlying marked skeletal discrepancy becoming apparent.

Surprisingly, some adult patients may still have an untreated reverse overjet associated with a displacement. Correction with a removable appliance may still be appropriate.

Unfavourable factors

Skeletal pattern

Where there is no displacing activity, the underlying skeletal pattern will be a more definite class III, which may be due to over-development of the mandible, under-development of the maxilla, or a combination of both. The Frankfort mandibular planes angle is frequently high in the more severe skeletal III patterns and such patients are more likely to grow unfavourably during adolescence.

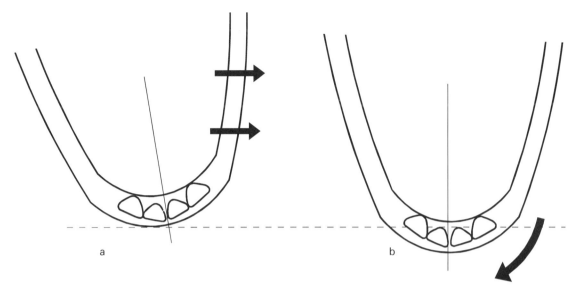

Figure 9.2 (a) A unilateral crossbite with a displacement of the mandible results in a centre-line shift. (b) Examination of the patient in the non-displaced position may demonstrate an underlying mild class III skeletal base.

Overbite and overjet

In the absence of a displacing activity and when the patient cannot readily obtain an edge-to-edge incisor relationship, successful correction is unlikely with removable appliances. Even when the patient is able to bite edge-to-edge, the prognosis will depend on the incisor inclination and the amount of overbite present. Where the overbite is reduced, the prospect for a stable long-term correction may be poor even if there is a mandibular displacement.

If the incisor inclination already compensates for the class III skeletal pattern (with the upper incisors proclined and the lower incisors retroclined), further labial movement of the upper incisors will often produce a traumatic relationship with the lower incisors. In such a situation it is unlikely that a stable incisor relationship can be achieved by orthodontic treatment alone.

Buccal crossbite

A unilateral crossbite can disguise an underlying class III skeletal pattern because the displacement causes the mandible to move slightly to one side on closure producing an effective shortening of its length. When the displacement is eliminated the mandible reverts to closure in centric and the prognathism is apparent (Figure 9.2). A unilateral crossbite with two or more incisors in reversed overjet is likely to be too difficult to correct with removable appliances.

A bilateral crossbite normally has to be accepted and may be an indication of an underlying skeletal pattern, which is too severe to respond to simple treatment.

Age factors

If a reversed overjet is present in the established permanent dentition the considerations of skeletal pattern, incisor angulation and displacement will be particularly important. In the pre-pubertal patient the possibility of further mandibular growth must be an important consideration.

A single, crowded, upper lateral incisor in crossbite, in the established dentition, may be difficult to correct with a removable appliance alone as these palatally placed incisors are usually associated with a centre-line shift (Figure 9.3).

Upper lateral incisors in lingual occlusion and with an increased overbite are frequently associated with an anterior displacement of the mandible on closure, due to a premature

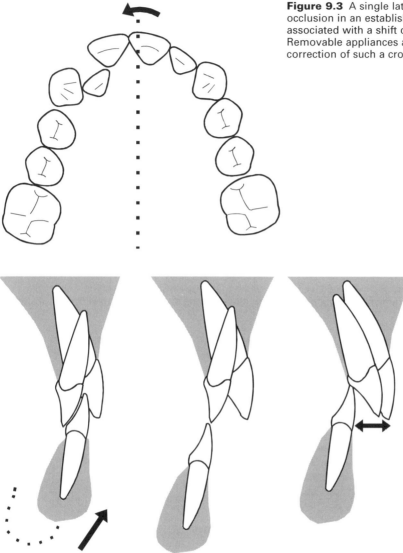

Figure 9.3 A single lateral incisor in lingual occlusion in an established dentition is often associated with a shift of the upper centre-line. Removable appliances alone cannot achieve correction of such a crossbite.

Figure 9.4 Upper lateral incisors, which are crowded palatally, may be associated with a forward displacement of the mandible on closure. (a) Examination of the patient with the lateral incisors in the initial contact position (b) may demonstrate a potentially increased overjet (c) in a case that initially appeared to be mild class III.

a   b   c

contact (Figure 9.4). It is important to check for this before treatment is started. Such a situation may disguise an underlying mild class II occlusion and correction may produce an increased overjet on the other incisors. Allowance may need to be made for this when planning treatment.

Patients with a skeletal III base, who present with upper lateral incisors in crossbite and with their apices palatally placed, will present particular difficulties. Teeth with this type of inclination are difficult to engage with

a spring to the palatal surface. Any forward movement is likely to reduce the overbite further and produce a very foreshortened appearance because of the forward inclination of the crowns. (A removable appliance may, however, still constitute a useful initial treatment phase.)

In the established dentition a mildly crowded lower arch, with incisor imbrication which will not improve spontaneously following extractions, renders treatment more difficult and usually necessitates the use of fixed appliances.

Aims of treatment

The aims of treatment are the correction of reverse overjet, alignment of the labial segments, elimination of any displacing activity and a stable result.

A critical factor in the stability of a corrected class III incisal relationship is the degree of overbite. The aim of treatment is generally to maintain the existing overbite and not to reduce it. Appliances should be designed to minimize overbite reduction. The use of molar capping to disengage the occlusion while a displacing activity is corrected has the advantage of inhibiting vertical growth of the posterior teeth and thus helping to maintain a positive overbite.

The proclination of an upper incisor will tend to reduce its vertical height and so to reduce the overbite (Figure 9.5). Because the upper incisor has a sloping palatal surface, a spring, which is designed to move the tooth forward, will also produce an intrusive component of force. The correct choice of spring or the use of a screw can minimize this.

Extraction considerations

In the mixed dentition stage, one or two incisors in crossbite are often associated with upper arch crowding. Extraction of the upper deciduous canines is often desirable to allow for temporary relief of upper labial segment crowding. Early correction can be worthwhile because it is more easily carried out before the eruption of successive teeth provides further obstruction. Such cases frequently require extraction of the lower deciduous canines to allow for some temporary relief of the lower incisor crowding, which assists any correction. It must be made clear to the parents that, ultimately, extraction of permanent teeth may be necessary.

In the established dentition, proclination of the upper incisors and expansion of the upper arch moves the teeth onto an arc of wider circumference, which effectively reduces crowding. Extractions may therefore need to be further back in the arch than in a class I or mild class II case with an equivalent degree of crowding. Where there is doubt, it may be wise to commence arch expansion, either anteroposteriorly or laterally, before deciding upon

extraction of permanent teeth. Residual extraction space towards the front of the arch may allow relapse of a corrected incisor position and because of this, first premolar extractions should only be considered when the crowding is marked. In the mildly crowded case, premolar extractions may be best avoided and the extraction of upper second molar teeth may sometimes be considered.

It is wise to be cautious about lower arch extractions. Where crowding is severe, the extraction of lower first premolars may be considered to relieve canine and incisor crowding, but in mildly crowded cases, fixed appliance treatment is indicated. Very occasionally,

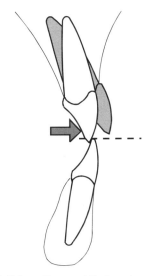

Figure 9.5 Where the overbite is reduced, proclination of the upper incisors will result in a further reduction in overbite and may produce an unstable incisor relationship.

extraction of a lower incisor may be appropriate; particularly if, as a result of a crossbite, it is labially displaced with reduced buccal bone and gingival recession. In such a case specialist advice should be sought.

In the upper arch, in some very crowded cases, with the canines forward and labial to the lateral incisors, it may be possible to extract a totally excluded lateral incisor and allow the canine to erupt into contact with the central incisor. Again, specialist advice should be sought before proceeding with such a plan.

Appliance design

Molar capping may assist by disengaging the occlusion and eliminating any displacing activity of the mandible on closure. This will usually require only a very thin layer of acrylic on the posterior teeth. Indeed, the cusp tips of the molars may perforate the acrylic. An anterior bite plane is usually contraindicated because it may reduce the overbite. An increase in overbite is often advantageous for a stable result.

Springs to move the upper incisors over the bite should avoid intrusive forces as far as possible. A 'T' spring inevitably has this effect so it is better to use a cranked cantilever spring. A double coil 'Z' spring can also be used – especially where space is limited – but is more difficult to adjust.

A unilateral buccal crossbite with a displacement is often associated with a single lateral incisor in lingual occlusion on the same side. Correction of the crossbite may be carried out with a removable appliance incorporating a mid-line screw to expand the upper arch. Molar capping is desirable to disengage the occlusion and eliminate the displacement. A cranked palatal finger spring can be incorporated to deal with the instanding incisor.

Retention must be adequate because the forces used to move the upper incisors forwards will, through their action on the inclined palatal surfaces of these teeth, cause a displacing force on the appliance. Retention is often poor in young children where the molar eruption is incomplete, but the presence of molar capping can help to retain the appliance. Where two or more incisors are to be moved over the bite, it can be useful to choose an appliance with a screw, which engages the labial segment. This has the advantage of providing additional retention at the front of the arch and further resisting displacement.

An appliance for lateral expansion and correction of lateral incisor in crossbite (Figure 9.6)

Active components
Screw, cranked palatal finger spring.

Anchorage
The arch is to be expanded symmetrically so anchorage is reciprocal.

Baseplate
The baseplate is split in the mid-line to allow for expansion. Posterior bite planes are required: (a) to prevent occlusal interference and eliminate the displacement; (b) to avoid secondary expansion of the lower arch by occlusal forces; and (c) to help seat the appliance, particularly after activation.

Points to note
The screw should be opened by the patient one-quarter turn per week. If the appliance is adjusted more frequently it may not seat fully and will become difficult to wear. After the expansion has been completed the molar capping should be removed and retention is

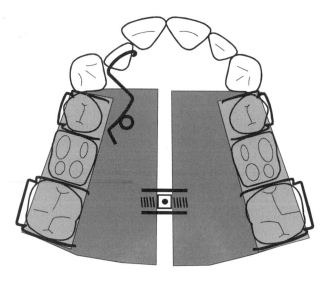

Figure 9.6 An appliance to expand the upper arch and correct a crossbite on 2|. Adams' clasps 64|46, cranked palatal finger spring (0.6 mm). A mid-line screw and molar capping.

continued for at least 3 months. The screw can be covered with cold-cured acrylic to prevent any unwanted movement.

An appliance to procline an instanding incisor (Figure.9.7)

Active component
A double cantilever spring may be used (see Figure 3.14, p. 20). For a narrow tooth, such as a lateral incisor, such springs are rather stiff and their range of action is limited, although this can be partly overcome by the use of 0.35 mm wire. (If two adjacent teeth are instanding, it is often preferable to use a single spring to procline both.) Alternatively, a cranked single cantilever spring may be suitable, because the crank keeps the spring clear of the other teeth. The coil should be positioned as far forward as possible or the direction of action may be incorrect. Both types of spring may be protected by being boxed-in under the baseplate, but as the tooth moves forward, full protection will be lost. This may allow a double cantilever spring to slip occlusally but a cranked finger spring will still be supported by the baseplate.

Retention
Most springs will displace the anterior part of the appliance and so, where possible, teeth in addition to the first molar should be clasped. In the mixed dentition such teeth will be deciduous canines or deciduous first molars, which do not offer good retention. In the older patient, canines or first premolars may be clasped.

Anchorage
The anchorage provided by the clasped teeth is more than adequate.

Baseplate
A bite plane will serve to clear the overbite while the incisors are being proclined. Normally, posterior bite planes should be used and are best trimmed so that there is about 1 mm clearance in the incisor area.

The elimination of occlusal contacts will help lower incisor irregularities to improve spontaneously. A slight lingual movement of the most prominent lower incisors means that the upper incisor has only to be proclined by a very small amount.

Points to note
Provided that the tooth is palatally inclined and the overbite is adequate, this is one of the simplest tooth movements and will normally be completed within a few weeks. Where there is a positive overbite, retention may not be necessary. An instanding incisor may, however, be only one feature of a more complex malocclusion and a complete case assessment must be performed before treatment is started. Where there is no positive overbite, or where the incisor apex is palatally displaced, treatment with a removable appliance may be unsatisfactory.

If the skeletal pattern is too severe further labial movement of the upper incisors will often produce a traumatic relationship with the

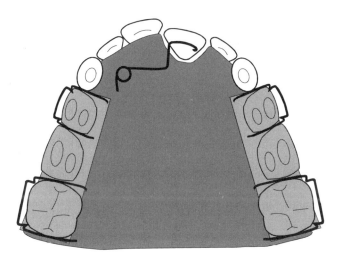

Figure 9.7 An appliance to procline 1̲. A cantilever spring (0.5 mm), Adams' clasps 6̲|6̲ (0.7 mm) and on D̲|D̲ (0.6 mm). Molar capping to disengage the occlusion.

lowers. As with a single instanding incisor, correction will not be stable unless there is a positive overbite at the end of treatment.

An appliance to procline the upper labial segment (Figure 9.8)

Active component
Double cantilever springs (or cranked finger springs, as described for single instanding incisors) can be used. In this case, $\underline{D|D}$ or $\underline{4|4}$ might be clasped to resist the displacing effect of the spring. When anterior retention is a problem a screw can be used (Figure 9.9). This has the advantage of being simple for the patient to manage and allowing retention to be improved by clasping the central incisors.

Retention
Clasps on $\underline{6|6}$ and $\underline{1|1}$ with a screw to move the labial segment forwards.

Anchorage
The teeth that are clasped provide adequate anchorage.

Baseplate
Posterior bite planes are used to clear the occlusion in the incisor region by about 1 mm. Where a screw is used, the baseplate is split.

Points to note
Patients sometimes find a screw positioned at the front of the mouth to be rather bulky. The patient is instructed to turn the screw one quarter-turn per week.

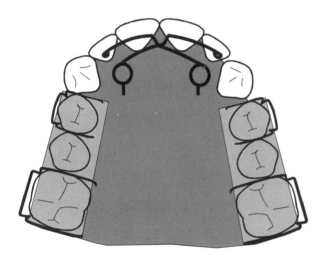

Figure 9.8 An appliance to procline the upper labial segment. Adams' clasps $\underline{64|46}$ (0.7 mm), palatal cantilever springs (0.6 mm) and molar capping.

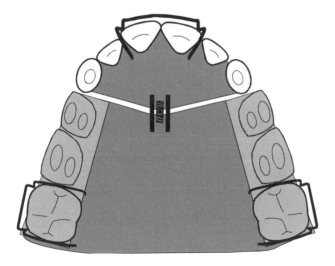

Figure 9.9 An appliance to procline $\underline{21|12}$. Adams' clasps $\underline{6|6}$ (0.7 mm), double Adams' clasps on $\underline{1|1}$ (0.7 mm), molar capping and a screw to procline $\underline{21|12}$.

Retention

The necessary length of retention will depend upon the depth of overbite at the completion of treatment. A corrected incisor crossbite with increased overbite at the end of treatment may require little or no retention. The first stage of retention in most cases will be to remove the molar capping. At the following visit the patient is instructed to wear the appliance on a nights-only basis for a further 2 months.

Where the overbite is reduced, retention should be maintained for longer. If a screw or springs have been used to correct the incisors and the overbite is reduced, it is often advisable to make a separate retainer such as a conventional appliance with a 'U' loop labial bow – specifically to hold the incisors in their new position. Where this seems unnecessary, it is possible to make the previous appliance passive by the addition of cold-cured acrylic, either to cover palatal springs and contact the incisors, or to lock a screw into the open position.

In some cases, particularly a lingually occluding lateral incisor, it is possible to increase the overbite and to reduce reliance on the retainers by adding composite to the incisal edge of the incisor to help maintain the corrected overjet.

Further reading

Nerder, P.H., Bakke, M., Solow, B. (1999) The functional shift of the mandible in unilateral posterior crossbite. *European Journal of Orthodontics*, **21**: 155–166

Ninou, S., Stephens, C.D. (1994) The early treatment of posterior crossbite – current understanding of continuing controversies. *Dental Update*, **21**: 420–426

Stephens, C.D., Jenkins, C.G.B. (1988) Crown modification using composite resin to achieve incisor overbite. *British Journal of Orthodontics*, **4**: 121–122

Chapter 10

Chairside management

It is at the beginning of treatment that the foundations of the future success of treatment are laid. Chairside management begins with assessment of the patient and formulation of a treatment plan, which should be clearly written down and should include the aims of treatment, the stages of treatment and any necessary extractions. The intended retention regimen should also be included.

It is at this stage that patient commitment and motivation must be assessed. Failure to appreciate possible problems and to discuss them with the patient can prejudice the future cooperation. A badly designed or constructed appliance will be difficult to wear and can undermine the cooperation of even the most enthusiastic patient.

Records

Good records are essential at the start of any treatment, both as an aid in the initial diagnosis and treatment planning and also to serve as a reference point during treatment.

Study models

Well-trimmed current study models are most important (Figure 10.1). The impressions should be taken using trays with deep flanges or

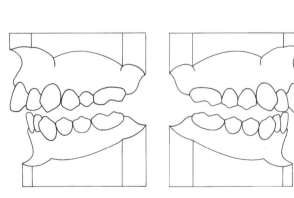

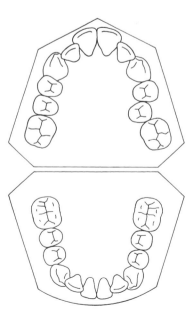

Figure 10.1 Well-trimmed study models.

built up with wax to ensure that the full depth of the buccal sulcus is reproduced. This enables the form of the alveolar process to be assessed. The models should be cast with adequate bases, the upper being trimmed symmetrically about the medial palatal raphe and the lower correspondingly. This ensures that any asymmetry of the arches will be recognized. The posterior surfaces of the models are trimmed flush so that the models can be related in occlusion by laying them backs-down on a flat surface. At the visit following the taking of the impressions, the models should be checked to ensure that the occlusion is correctly recorded with the mandible in centric relation. If there is any doubt about the articulation of the models the correct position should be registered by drawing a vertical pencil line through the occlusion of the molars on both sides and the models returned to the laboratory for re-trimming.

Radiographs

Good radiographic records are necessary to confirm the position of any unerupted teeth and the condition of the alveolar bones. This is obviously important before deciding upon the choice of teeth for extraction, but it may also be useful in the event of untoward damage to the teeth during treatment. The normal radiograph would be a dental pantomogram (DPT). Should there be any doubt about the condition of the incisors or any possibility of supernumerary teeth being present, the DPT is supplemented with an intraoral occlusal view of the upper incisor region. An alternative method is to use rotated lateral oblique radiographs (bimolars) and a standard occlusal of the upper anterior region.

For the majority of cases that are suitable for treatment with removable appliances lateral skull radiographs are not essential. Where limited tooth movement is being carried out and all successional teeth have erupted, it may be possible, in some circumstances, to carry out treatment without radiographs.

Photographs

Photographs form an important record of the patient's occlusion and appearance. Intraoral photographs should include an anterior view and right and left buccal views with the teeth in occlusion. Extraoral views should show full face and profile.

One advantage of intraoral photographs is that they will demonstrate any possible decalcification or hypoplastic marks which are present at the start of treatment which may be a useful record in case of any questions arising at the end of treatment.

Equipment

The following equipment is required for adjustment of a removable appliance.

Wire bending pliers

Adams' universal pliers (with tips impregnated with tungsten carbide) are the most useful in the adjustment of appliances (Figure 10.2). Spring forming pliers are also useful (Figure 10.3).

Different manufacturers produce pliers with varying handle shapes and sizes. Find a pair that feels comfortable before you buy them.

Reserve the plier tips for adjusting the lighter wires and springs. Where heavy gauge wires (for example extraoral facebows) require

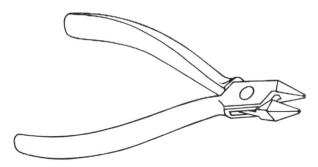

Figure 10.2 Adams' universal pliers.

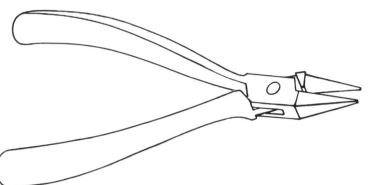

Figure 10.3 Spring forming pliers.

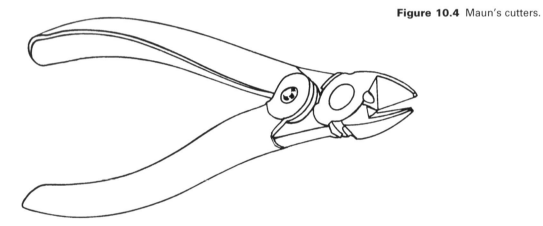

Figure 10.4 Maun's cutters.

Figure 10.5 Spring dividers.

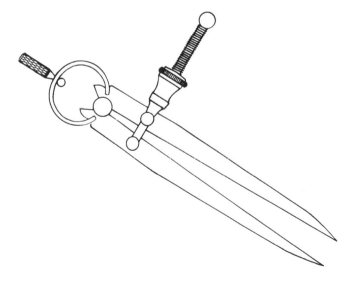

adjustment, grasp the wire closer to the hinge to avoid damage.

Maun cutting pliers

These are a robust pair of wire cutting pliers, which will be suitable for cutting stainless steel wires of the dimensions commonly used for removable appliances (Figure 10.4). If these are not available a pair of wire cutters that can cut wire up to 1.25 mm in diameter will be needed.

Measuring instruments

A pair of stainless steel spring dividers enables the distances between teeth to be measured (Figure 10.5) and a 15 cm rule in millimetre divisions is useful for measuring overjet and treatment changes.

Fitting a new removable appliance

A removable appliance does not always need to be fitted immediately after teeth have been extracted. In many cases it is possible to allow spontaneous tooth movement to occur for a month or more before the appliance is needed. In other cases, where the space available for tooth movement is barely sufficient, the appliance should be fitted before the extractions are carried out. If there is any doubt about the patient's cooperation it is good practice to fit the appliance and let it be worn for a time prior to the extractions.

- The appliance should have been designed at the time of taking the impression and with the patient still in the chair. It can represent false economy to attempt to move too many teeth with one appliance. Treatment will be better controlled and more rapidly completed if a separate appliance is used for each group of tooth movements. If up-to-date study models already exist, then only a single impression for a working model is required – otherwise an upper and lower impression may be taken to provide study models and a duplicate of the relevant model for appliance construction. The impressions must be checked to ensure that there are no drags or large air bubbles and also to be sure that the impression material is well extended and fully attached to the tray.

  The appliance should be fitted within 1 or 2 weeks after the impression has been taken.
- At the time of fitting pick up the appliance and run the fingers over the baseplate – particularly the fitting surface – checking for any sharp areas. Air bubbles on the model can produce roughness of the acrylic but such areas can be quickly smoothed, as can any sharp ends of wire.
- Show the appliance to the patient and demonstrate the retaining clasps and active springs, drawing attention to the need to take care not to distort any of the active parts of the appliance during its insertion and removal.

Retention

This should always be checked carefully. If the appliance is well made little adjustment will be necessary. It should snap easily into place with finger pressure and be a firm fit, although readily removable. Retention may be poor because the appliance is badly designed to resist the displacing forces to which it is subjected. Attention to design should avoid this.

Adjustment of clasps

Clasps made according to Adams' design offer good retention. Frequently, however, the operator is presented with an appliance on which the clasps are faulty and adjustments may be necessary.

When adjusting clasps the operator should avoid, as far as possible, bending the wire at points where it has already been bent during construction by the technician. The only exception to this rule is that where the clasps are initially too tight to permit insertion, it may be necessary to grip each arrowhead in turn with the pliers and bend it outwards (Figure 10.6). Once the appliance can be seated (if necessary with the support of a finger) the accurate positioning of the arrowheads can be investigated. Possible faults are as follows:

Horizontal

The arrowheads do not contact the tooth or else grip it too tightly.

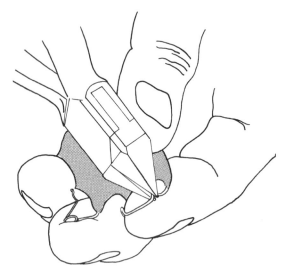

Figure 10.6 Occasionally it is necessary to bend the arrowhead of an Adams' clasp.

Vertical

The arrowheads grip too far occlusally or else push up into the gingivae.

These faults can be corrected in most cases by a combination of bends at two points (Figure 10.7). Bending the wire just beyond the point where it has passed over the embrasure controls its vertical position. Bending it nearer to the arrowhead controls its bucco-lingual position.

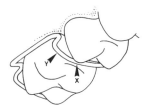

Figure 10.7 The fit of a clasp can be adjusted by bending the wire at two points. Adjustment at X moves the arrowhead vertically; adjustment at Y moves it horizontally.

Take as an example a clasp that is found to have an arrowhead pushing into the gingivae (Figure 10.8a). The wire can be bent at point X to move the arrowhead occlusally (Figure 10.8b). The height will be corrected but the adjustment will also have the effect of moving the arrowhead away from the tooth. A bend can then be placed at point Y to compensate for this (Figure 10.8c).

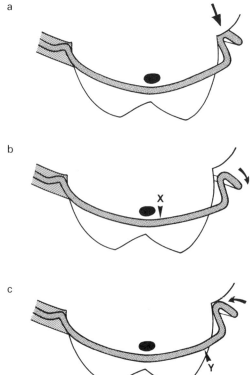

Figure 10.8 (a) The arrowhead is pushing into the gingival margin. (b) First adjustment at point X moves the arrowhead away from the tooth. (c) Second adjustment restores tooth contact with the arrowhead at the correct height.

If the arrowhead grips too far occlusally it can be moved buccally by an adjustment at point Y. A further adjustment at point X will then bring it into contact at the correct position (Figure 10.9).

It is important that the clasp does not grip the tooth too tightly and an undercut of 0.25 mm has been shown to give an adequate clasp. It is useless to attempt to tighten the clasp by bending the wire at the point where it emerges from the acrylic. This will merely interfere with the passage of the wire across the embrasure and prevent full seating of the appliance. The only indication for adjustment at this point occurs in a case where the wire passes high over the embrasure and interferes with the occlusion.

Poor retention may be due to a conically shaped tooth, which offers little undercut. This is especially common when second molars are being clasped.

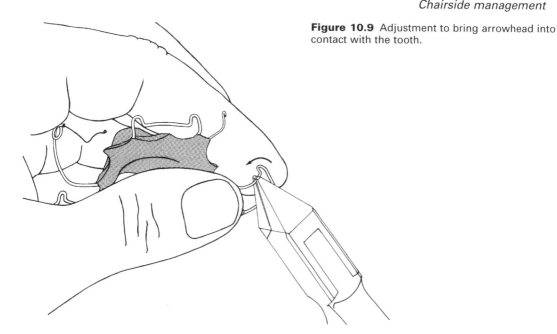

Figure 10.9 Adjustment to bring arrowhead into contact with the tooth.

Adjustments to the acrylic

On occasion, slight initial trimming may be necessary to allow insertion, but beyond this, some adjustments to the baseplate may also be necessary. The acrylic will need to be trimmed to permit active tooth movement. This is of great importance but is frequently overlooked. The appliance should be inspected *in situ* to ensure that no part of the acrylic contacts the tooth to be moved and that this tooth movement will not result in contact before the next visit. It is also sensible to trim the acrylic so that any desired passive movement might occur, for example to permit a buccally placed canine to move into line as a premolar is being retracted.

Bite planes

Any excessive thickness may need to be reduced and bite planes adjusted to give even contacts. In the case of posterior bite planes, careful trimming will usually be necessary to ensure that the occlusion is evenly distributed. An anterior bite plane will need to be undermined on an appliance designed to reduce an overjet before activating the labial spring.

Adjustment to active wirework

The appliance should now be easy to fit and have adequate retention. Before activating springs the labial wires, loops and buccal springs should be adjusted if necessary so that they lie at the correct height and do not traumatize the cheeks, lips and gingivae.

During the first few days with a new appliance the patient has to get used to inserting it correctly, must adapt to its presence and perhaps put up with a mild degree of discomfort. It is sensible to provide only very light activation so that the appliance is self-activating and the springs cannot readily slip into the wrong position. This will imply activation of about 1 mm for a palatal spring and 0.5 mm for a 0.7 mm buccal spring. It will often not be possible to position a palatal spring close to the gingival margin at the first visit because of contact with the neighbouring tooth. This can be corrected at the next visit when some movement should have taken place.

Demonstration to the patient

- Show the patient the appliance in the mouth using a mirror, demonstrating how it should be inserted and removed. (During fitting, any anterior clasp on the incisors will generally be engaged and the position of the springs checked before upward pressure is applied to the palatal acrylic with a finger or thumb (Figure 10.10). Removal should be achieved by exerting finger pressure on the

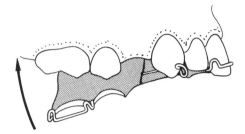

Figure 10.10 Correct method of insertion of an appliance. Engage the anterior clasp first; press the acrylic pad upwards until the molar clasps engage. Removal is accomplished by pulling down on the molar clasps.

bridges of the Adams' clasps on the first molars to disengage them before the front of the appliance is disengaged.)

• Allow the patient to remove and replace the appliance in front of you.

• Check that the appliance has been seated correctly, paying particular attention to the position of active springs after the patient has inserted it.

The patient should be instructed to wear the appliance full time, i.e. all day, all night, for meals and, as far as possible, for sports. Wear during meals is especially important, particularly if bite opening has to be achieved or if the teeth are being moved across the bite. As far as possible, cleaning should be carried out after meals and particular care should be given to cleaning the fitting surface of the appliance, either with a nail brush or with the patient's own tooth brush. If, on occasion, circumstances do not permit this then the appliance should at least be removed from the mouth and rinsed under a tap. If it does prove necessary to remove the appliance from the mouth other than for cleaning, for example during contact sports or the playing of a wind instrument, the patient should be instructed to keep the appliance in a small, rigid box which will protect it from accidental damage.

Initially the patient will be very aware of the large bulk of the appliance and may experience excess salivation and difficulty in swallowing. Reassurance should be given that this is quite normal and that the appliance will rapidly feel more comfortable. Difficulties with excessive salivation and swallowing usually disappear within a few hours. Normal speech may take 24 to 48 hours to achieve. The most difficult adap-tation is to accept the wear of the appliance at meal times and this may take several days to accomplish. The patient should be encouraged to persevere until this has been achieved.

Information

The patient should be given simple verbal instructions:

• Sticky sweets must be avoided. Chewing gum – other than one especially formulated for denture wearers – will adhere to the acrylic. Good oral hygiene is important – keeping the appliance and the mouth clean.

• If the appliance breaks or causes discomfort or trauma to the cheeks or tongue, the patient should not wait for a routine visit but contact the practice for an earlier appointment. The patient should continue to wear the appliance for some hours each day if possible to maintain its fit. If the appliance cannot be worn it should be kept moist.

• Where the patient is a child, the parent should be brought into the surgery so that the instructions can be repeated. This not only informs the parent but also allows reinforcement of the instructions to the child.

• A printed information sheet on the use of the appliance should be given to the patient to take home (Appendix 2).

• A further appointment should be made for the patient to be seen in approximately 2–3 weeks' time.

It is important that in the event of breakage, trauma to soft tissue or discomfort, the patient should be seen at the earliest opportunity – so that wear is not interrupted. The patient should be given some soft wax when the appliance is fitted. A small piece of the wax placed over a wire, which is causing irritation, may improve the comfort until a surgery visit is possible.

The printed instruction sheet should not be handed over until after verbal instruction has been given. This encourages the patient to concentrate on the instructions without being distracted.

Difficulty in fitting an appliance

There are several reasons why a new appliance may not fit.

The wrong appliance

In a busy practice or laboratory incorrect labelling can occur. It is possible that the wrong appliance has been returned.

Anticipation of extractions

If the technician has removed from the model the teeth which are to be extracted, and the appliance encroaches on this area, it will not fit without modification until the extractions have been carried out. The technician should be asked to leave all existing teeth on the model during appliance construction, except in cases where wires are to be positioned across extraction spaces.

Eruption of teeth

The eruption of palatally placed teeth, particularly upper second premolars, can cause problems. This usually occurs when there has been a delay in fitting the appliance since the impression was taken. Unless the embedded parts of the wirework override the erupting teeth, the acrylic can be trimmed away, but if the wirework is in the way, this provides a considerable difficulty. The eruption of an instanding tooth should be anticipated when designing the appliance.

Inadequate impression

An impression, which has been removed from the mouth before it is completely set, which has come away from the tray or been allowed to dry out, will be distorted. Any appliance made on the model from such an impression is unlikely to fit well. Similarly, inadequately extended impressions or those with air blows of any size may present problems which the technician cannot overcome.

Delay since the impression

Forward movement of the buccal segments following orthodontic extractions or natural loss of deciduous teeth may interfere with fitting. This is very common when first molars have been extracted.

Excessive undercut

Undercuts rarely give rise to a problem in the upper arch but can prevent a lower appliance from seating properly. Such undercuts need to be blocked out on the model before the appliance is made, because subsequent trimming may weaken the appliance unduly.

Wire loops, which lie close to the gingivae, take no account of the path of insertion so that they may impinge on the mucosa as the appliance is seated. Careful adjustment of the appliance can usually avoid this.

Difficulties with clasps

Check the design of the Adams' clasps and ensure that there is adequate undercut on the first molars. Overtrimming of the model during construction can make the clasps so tight that insertion is impossible. In adult patients, trimming is usually unnecessary and even to take the arrowheads up to the gingivae may mean that excessive undercut is engaged.

Subsequent appliances

Occasionally a subsequent appliance will not fit because movement of the teeth has occurred since the impression was taken. This may result because the previous appliance was left active or because the patient has ceased to wear it. Either of these events can cause inconvenience and the latter can even produce the situation where neither the new nor the old appliance will fit.

Subsequent visits

Successful management of orthodontic treatment depends upon careful assessment at each visit so that lack of progress or unwanted tooth movements can be recognized early and remedial action is taken. The appliance must be adjusted with care and good records need to be kept.

The patient should be seen 2 or 3 weeks after the appliance has been fitted and then at monthly intervals. Inadequate attention to detail at regular visits may mean that something is overlooked and that progress is slow or erratic. The acrylic or the occlusion may interfere with tooth movement, unintended movements may be taking place or anchorage loss may be occurring. Oral hygiene can also deteriorate, unnoticed, over the course of a few visits.

General practitioners should try to set aside some 'protected time' by reserving a particular session for orthodontic work. It is when the 'quick orthodontic adjustment' is sandwiched between time-consuming restorative or surgical procedures that inadequate thought and attention are so often given.

Preliminary discussion with the patient

- Enquire whether the patient has experienced any problems with the appliance since the previous visit. Avoid leading questions such as 'Have you been wearing the appliance?' This merely encourages an affirmative answer, even if the patient has not been cooperating. The operator should be alert for any signs of poor cooperation. For example, it is generally a bad sign if the appliance is not actually in the mouth, even if the patient claims that it had been removed for cleaning before entering the surgery. Poor speech is also often a symptom of poor wear (but do check that this is not the patient's normal voice before making accusations).
- Look into the mouth before the appliance is removed. The fit of the appliance is then easily assessed. Similarly, it is easy to see whether it is being correctly worn and whether all springs are correctly positioned. Excessive looseness may lead the operator to suspect that the patient has developed the habit of moving the appliance up and down with the tongue. This is a sure method of producing multiple fractures of wire during treatment and must be firmly discouraged.
- If you conclude that the appliance has not been worn as directed, raise the matter directly: 'Why have you been leaving your brace out?'

The operator should then remove the appliance noting any degree of activation remaining in the springs. The fitting surface of the appliance will give some clue to oral hygiene but in addition the teeth, gingivae and oral mucosa, particularly the area covered by the appliance, should be inspected. Generalized palatal inflammation may reflect the need for more thorough oral hygiene. Heaping up of the gingivae around the teeth being moved indicates that the appliance has not been trimmed away adequately.

Changes in the occlusion since the last visit

It is good practice to measure and record changes in tooth position at each visit rather than simply entering a verbal comment. A simple measurement is often sufficient, for example during retraction of upper canines a pair of dividers may be used to measure the distance from the highest part of the buccal fissure of the first molar to the tip of the canine (Figure 10.11). The distance between the points of the dividers can then be measured and recorded in the patient's folder.

Measurements are usually possible for any tooth movement. When distal movement of upper molars is being carried out, a measurement from the buccal fissure of the first molar to the mesial corner of the central incisor will be of use and during lateral arch expansion measurement across specified cusps will serve. Overjet reduction can be measured by means of a ruler with a millimetre scale, with the zero point at the extreme end. It should be pointed out that overjet measurement is an arbitrary, rather than a defined, parameter and represents the horizontal distance between the labial surface of the lower incisor and the incisal edge of the uppers. Some variation is bound to occur as a result of different inclinations of the ruler but in practice this is small and the overjet measurement is reproducible. The operator should get into the habit of using the same points of reference as a routine, for example overjet measurements might be taken from the

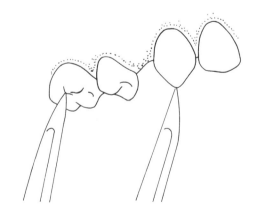

Figure 10.11 Measurement to assess canine retraction. This must be combined with a record of overjet to ensure that anchorage loss is not occurring.

tip of the upper left central incisor. When this routine must be changed, perhaps because the tooth in question is fractured or lost, then the position from which the measurements are taken should be recorded carefully in the notes.

Anchorage

Newton's third law of motion tells us that every force has an equal and opposite reaction. When teeth are being moved the reactive force will be transmitted through the appliance and will affect other teeth which are themselves capable of movement. Measurements such as those described above indicate that movement is taking place but do not show that only the intended teeth are moving. It is important to take further measurements at each visit to confirm that anchorage loss is not occurring.

- Where only one arch is being treated it is usually easy to use the other arch as a reference. In the case of upper canine retraction a measurement of overjet should be taken (Figure 10.12) and any increase in this is usually a warning that anchorage is being lost (Figure 10.13). The molar relationship will also become more class II. When lower arch extractions have been carried out assessment can become more difficult.
- Imbricated lower incisors can align spontaneously and if the overjet was measured from a tooth which had been prominent it will appear to increase as this alignment occurs.
- Where headgear is being worn it is useful to ask the patient to keep a diary of wear. By giving the patient a target number of hours to be achieved per week, motivation can be

improved. It is important to ask to see the diary at each visit and to give encouragement or praise in order to reinforce the patient's efforts. Where cooperation is not adequate, all that can be done is to emphasize to the patient (and parent) that failure to wear the appliance as instructed can only delay treatment and prejudice the result.

- Where marked anchorage loss has occurred, changes in the relationship of the two arches will become noticeable. If the upper teeth are brought forward during the canine retraction they will retain the previous archwidth because they are held by the baseplate. They will therefore tend to become buccally placed.

When unwanted movement is discovered, corrective action should be taken at once. If the active components are exerting too great a force this must be reduced. Space requirements should be reassessed. If there is space to spare some loss of anchorage may be accepted. If space is short, however, anchorage reinforcement, usually with headgear, is essential.

Lack of satisfactory progress

Is the tooth free to move?

If the baseplate is in contact with the tooth it should be cut away sufficiently to ensure that further obstruction does not occur. Where the obstruction is due to occlusal interference the bite plane may need to be thickened by the addition of cold-cured acrylic. Make certain that an unerupted tooth or retained root has not been overlooked.

Has the correct force been applied?

Check that a spring is located correctly and on the right side of the tooth when the patient inserts the appliance. Make sure that the spring is adequately activated. Where a screw-plate is being used the patient may be adjusting the screw incorrectly. The operator can ask the patient to demonstrate turning and the screw can be turned back to check that the number of turns corresponds with that expected.

The use of heavy pressures will cause hyalinization within the periodontal ligament and delay resorption, so light pressure should be maintained and the patient should be warned

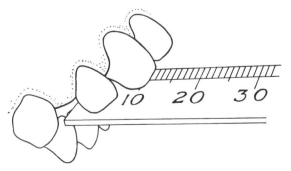

Figure 10.12 Measurement of overjet using a millimetre steel rule.

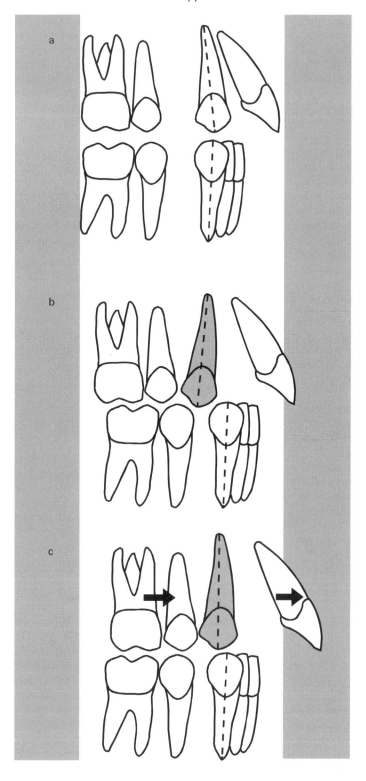

Figure 10.13 Assessment of anchorage during canine retraction. (a) Initial occlusion. (b) Correct forces have been used and the appliance worn as instructed. 3| has been retracted into a satisfactory class I relationship with 3| with little increase in overjet. (c) Anchorage loss is demonstrated. No further retraction of 3| is possible as the posterior teeth have moved forwards and the overjet has increased. It will not now be possible to reduce the overjet fully.

that treatment will be lengthy. In very rare cases, treatment may be prolonged by the presence of dense alveolar bone. Although the problem is rare, a similar situation can arise where a tooth, often an upper canine, is buccally displaced into the cortical plate. The bone surrounding the root is dense and lamellar and if the tooth is moved parallel to the line of the arch progress will be slow. Such a tooth should be moved into the line of the arch by the shortest path and then retracted through the cancellous bone of the alveolar process.

Has the appliance been worn as instructed?

Provided that the appliance has been correctly adjusted lack of tooth movement is usually due to inadequate wear. It is sensible to look for other signs of poor wear before discussing this with the patient. Difficulty in handling and inserting the appliance, speech problems, poor fit, lack of attrition facets on bite planes and an absence of marks on the palate at the periphery of the baseplate – all these point to lack of full-time wear. Careful questioning of the patient may elicit that it is left out for meals, at night, or at school.

Activation

For a single rooted tooth a force of 30–40 g is appropriate to produce controlled movement with minimal tipping. The thickness and length of the spring will determine the amount of activation necessary to produce such a force, but a desirable activation is roughly one-third to one-half a unit (about 3 or 4 mm). A palatal finger spring constructed in 0.5 mm wire correctly activated will deliver the desired force (Figure 10.14). If more activation is attempted the appliance may be difficult to insert correctly. The chance of the spring being wrongly positioned is increased and the spring is also more prone to damage.

A thicker or shorter spring may easily produce a force that is too heavy. For example, if a buccal canine retractor is constructed in 0.7 mm wire, activation must not be more than a third of the width of the canine to keep the force below 40 g. The tooth will quickly move through this distance and halt. Unless the patient attends frequently this produces slow movement and

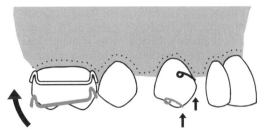

Figure 10.14 Correct degree of activation of a canine spring. The spring should just contact the mesial incline on the canine before full insertion of the appliance.

provides a temptation to overactivate the appliance. This may result in pain, anchorage slip and perhaps unwanted tilting of the tooth.

In general, palatal finger springs made to the design described are ideal and we favour the use of these whenever possible. If the operator has access to a force gauge of the 'Correx' type (Figure 10.15), it is possible to check the spring pressure being applied. This may be carried out in the following manner:

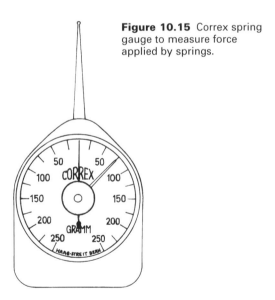

Figure 10.15 Correx spring gauge to measure force applied by springs.

Palatal springs

- The appliance is placed in the mouth with the spring in the correct position. The point at the edge of the acrylic from which the spring emerges is marked with a wax pencil. The point on the spring that delivers the force to the tooth should also be marked.

- The appliance is withdrawn from the mouth.
- The arm of the force gauge can then be pushed against the spring to return it to the mark on the baseplate. The force that will be delivered to the tooth can then be read.

Buccal springs

A buccal spring can be checked by measuring the position of the spring tip relative to the mesial arrowhead of the molar clasp on that side. This can be done with a pair of spring dividers when the appliance is in the mouth. The appliance is removed from the mouth and the arm of the force gauge again used to flex the spring back into its original place.

It is not necessary to measure force routinely in this manner, but it does help the operator to assess the amount of activation that will deliver the required force. Once this activation has been assessed it is still often useful to mark the position of a palatal spring with a wax pencil when the appliance is in position. The position of a buccal spring can be measured in the way described so that the actual amount of activation can be seen more easily.

Buccal canine retraction springs

Activation is carried out by holding the spring close to the coil with the plier beaks and flexing it with a finger or thumb until the desired position is reached. During activation the spring is permanently deformed by bending it beyond its elastic limit. It is good practice to avoid bending the spring at places where the wire has been bent during its formation and also to avoid carrying out successive activations at the same position. It should be remembered that activation of a spring offers a chance to modify the direction of tooth movement.

An appliance may sometimes be constructed with the coils of the canine finger springs, for example, placed too far distally. Simple activation of the spring from the coil will move the canine buccally as it is retracted. A crank progressively placed into the spring will provide activation and help to limit this tendency. When such cranking is not necessary the bend should be placed near to the coil.

In the case of a buccal spring it may often be necessary to adjust the spring at more than one point. The wire can be bent near to where it emerges on the buccal side of the arch so that the coil is correctly positioned. The coil itself can then be grasped in the beaks of the spring forming pliers and the free end flexed with the thumb to the desired position.

Secondary adjustments

Both buccal and palatal springs may require further adjustment. In the case of a palatal finger spring, the height may need adjustment so that the spring rests just clear of the gingival margin. If the wire projects too far buccally it may cause trauma to the cheek and require shortening. If a guard is being used care must be taken to see that the spring slides smoothly.

A buccal spring may also require adjustment for height and it may be necessary to flex the free end of the spring inward with the thumb so that it engages the tooth firmly, or sometimes to flex the entire spring inwards if the coil is too prominent.

When such adjustments have been carried out it is necessary to re-check that the spring activation has not been inadvertently altered.

Labial wires

The general principle of avoiding existing bends during activation and of carrying out the adjustment at different points still applies. Where the incisors are irregular it may be necessary to combine careful selective grinding of the palatal acrylic with activation of the labial wire. The wire may also be kinked to bring pressure to bear on a particular tooth and so help in obtaining alignment.

Again, it is possible to measure activation of anterior wires and this can be done by drilling a small pin-hole into the acrylic of the anterior bite plane and measuring from this to the mid-point of the labial wire, which can be marked with a wax pencil. The difference between this measurement taken with the appliance in and out of the mouth will show the amount of activation (Figure 10.16). A spring gauge can be used to produce the same amount of deflection and so indicate the force being used.

The labial bow

This is activated by reducing the size of the loops. Each side is dealt with individually by

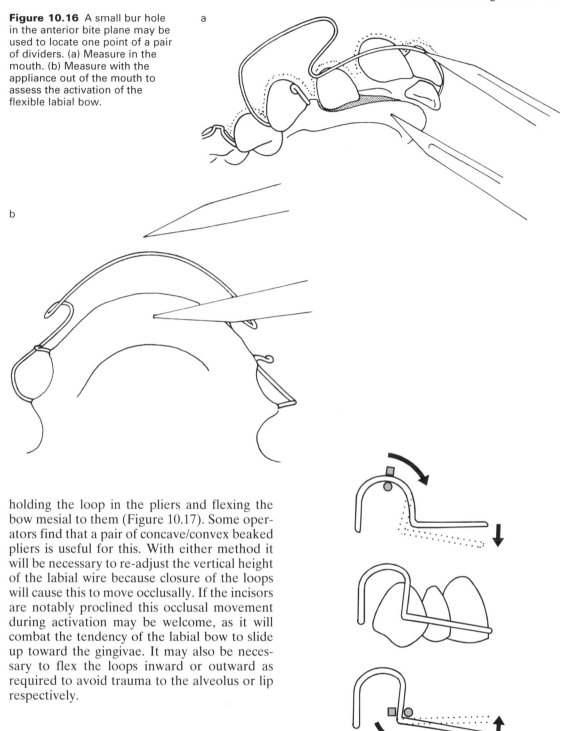

Figure 10.16 A small bur hole in the anterior bite plane may be used to locate one point of a pair of dividers. (a) Measure in the mouth. (b) Measure with the appliance out of the mouth to assess the activation of the flexible labial bow.

holding the loop in the pliers and flexing the bow mesial to them (Figure 10.17). Some operators find that a pair of concave/convex beaked pliers is useful for this. With either method it will be necessary to re-adjust the vertical height of the labial wire because closure of the loops will cause this to move occlusally. If the incisors are notably proclined this occlusal movement during activation may be welcome, as it will combat the tendency of the labial bow to slide up toward the gingivae. It may also be necessary to flex the loops inward or outward as required to avoid trauma to the alveolus or lip respectively.

Light wires

Light wires such as the apron spring and Roberts' retractor again need activation on each side. The wire should be gripped near to

Figure 10.17 Closure of a 'U' loop bow moves the bow incisally. A second adjustment is necessary to bring the bow onto the correct position on the labial face of the incisors.

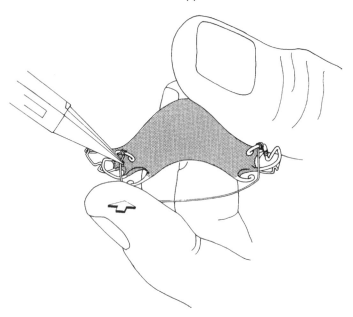

Figure 10.18 Activation of an apron spring. The procedure for a Roberts' retractor is identical.

the top of the descending vertical arm and the spring flexed palatally (Figure 10.18). Vertical adjustment is usually unnecessary but the supporting arms may again need bucco-palatal adjustment so that trauma is avoided.

Springs carrying out lingual movements

Buccal springs (described in Chapter 3) to move teeth palatally can be adjusted in a similar manner to that described for buccal canine springs. A buccal canine spring can itself be used to push a tooth palatally, perhaps at the end of retraction. To achieve this, the end of the spring, which engages the tooth, is bent through 90 degrees and the spring is adapted so that this can rest on the buccal face of the canine.

Springs carrying out buccal movement

Cranked palatal finger springs can be adjusted in the manner described for palatal finger springs. 'T' springs are useful for pushing premolars buccally and can be activated simply by seizing the cross-piece of the 'T' and pulling the spring outwards and slightly away from the fitting surface of the acrylic so that it binds on

the tooth during insertion. The provision of extra loops allows for further adjustment of the spring as the tooth moves.

'Z' springs are useful for proclining individual incisors. Again, the wire is gripped in the pliers and pulled forward and slightly upward from the acrylic to activate it (Figure 10.19). By flexing the spring in this manner the appliance is self-activating as it is put into the mouth and

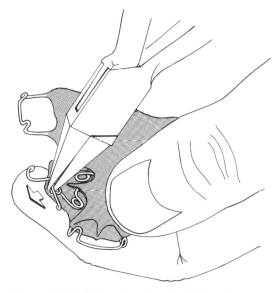

Figure 10.19 Activation of a palatal 'Z' spring.

any tendency for the spring to be trapped over the incisal edge of the tooth by the acrylic is avoided.

Acrylic

Adjustments to the acrylic may be required from time to time. At each visit it is important to check that the teeth being moved are free from contact with the acrylic and likely to remain so at least until the next appointment. When carrying out any trimming to accomplish this it must be remembered that allowance has to be made for the soft tissue which may be heaped up in advance of a moving tooth.

Anterior bite planes may need to be built up to continue bite opening or possibly to replace acrylic as a result of occlusal wear. During incisor retraction, acrylic will need to be trimmed from the fitting surface to permit tooth movement.

Posterior bite planes may need to be repaired during use as small fragments break away. They are trimmed to reduce the degree of bite opening as successful tooth movement occurs. Such reduction is usually carried out during two successive visits and precedes the total removal of the occlusal cover. Occasionally it may be possible to remove occlusal cover entirely at one appointment when a tooth in crossbite has corrected sufficiently to allow the posterior teeth into occlusion without trauma to the newly moved tooth.

General dental care

The state of the oral hygiene must be borne in mind at each appointment and any deficiency pointed out to the patient and corrected. It is also wise from time to time to check that the patient's visit to the general practitioner for routine inspections and treatment is being continued.

Further reading

Isaacson, K.G., Thom, A.R.T. (eds) (2001) *Orthodontic Radiographs – Guidelines*. British Orthodontic Society, London

Kerr, W.J.S. (1984) Appliance breakages. *British Journal of Orthodontics*, **11**: 137–142

Stewart, F.N., Kerr, W.J.S., Taylor, P.J.S. (1997) Appliance wear, the patient's point of view. *European Journal of Orthodontics*, **19**: 377–382

Chapter 11

Retainers

Orthodontics can only confer benefit to the patient if tooth movements that are achieved remain stable after treatment. A period of retention is always necessary after active treatment. In a few situations the corrected occlusion will provide its own retention (for example a corrected incisor, formerly in lingual occlusion, which has good, positive overbite) but usually a period of retention must be considered.

The aim of the retention phase is to ensure that the tooth movements that have been carried out are held while the periodontal fibres and the surrounding alveolar bone reorganize. Treatment usually aims to achieve a stable result, but the work of Little *et al.* (1988) has shown that crowding is a progressive condition which may continue to increase throughout life, with no identifiable predisposing factors. This is particularly marked in the lower labial segment and, even when the lower inter canine width has not been increased by treatment, lower incisor crowding may continue to increase. Patients should be made aware of this possibility and alerted to the fact that, even though orthodontic treatment may align the lower incisors, permanent retention will be necessary if perfect lower incisor alignment is to be guaranteed indefinitely.

At a time when retention times are tending to increase and more cases are being considered for permanent retention it might be asked whether extractions are necessary and whether treatment could not be limited to non-extraction alignment and permanent retention. We consider, however, that treatment should be based on the principle of the relief of crowding and that teeth should be placed in a position of stability before retention is commenced. It is physiologically unsound to hold teeth in an unstable position.

Removable retainers have an important part to play in all forms of orthodontic treatment and may be used following removable, fixed or functional appliance treatment.

Types of retainers

Converted appliance

The final removable appliance used during treatment can sometimes be converted into a retainer by deactivating any springs and adding cold-cured acrylic to make them passive and to lock any screws into position. The appliance can then be worn full time for 2–3 months before, if necessary, being worn only at night for a further 6 months. This type of retention might follow, for example, the correction of a lingual crossbite in the mixed dentition, which is frequently carried out with an upper removable appliance using springs or screws. If molar capping has been used it should be removed before the appliance is converted to a retainer. If the corrected incisor has an overbite of 2 mm or more the prognosis for stability is good, but if the overbite is reduced then the appliance should be converted to a retainer by the method described.

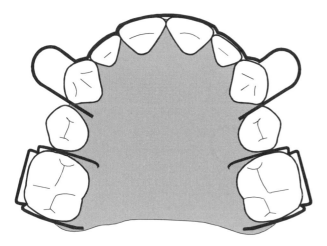

Figure 11.1 A Hawley retainer. Adams' clasps 6|6 (0.7 mm) and a fitted 'U' loop labial bow (0.7 mm).

'U' loop labial bow retainer (Hawley)

The appliance generally has Adams' clasps on the upper first molars and a 'U' loop labial bow lying against the incisors (Figure 11.1). The acrylic contacts the palatal surface of the teeth all the way around the arch. When fitting this type of retainer it is important that the labial bow contacts the incisors – especially any aspect of an incisor that may have been displaced at the start of the treatment. The acrylic should be in contact with the incisors unless an attempt is being made to achieve slight over-correction of a pre-existing rotation. In such a case, the acrylic may need to be trimmed adjacent to the most displaced part of a tooth.

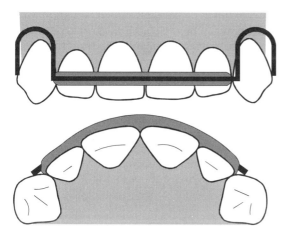

Figure 11.2 A modified bow retainer. The anterior part of the labial bow is covered in acrylic, which engages the embrasures between the incisors.

Acrylic covered labial bow

Labial bows have sometimes been made 'fitted', i.e. with the wire shaped to fit the labial contour of the incisors precisely. This is now more satisfactorily achieved by the addition of a narrow band of acrylic to the labial bow (Figure 11.2). This modification enables a more accurate fit than can be achieved with a labial bow alone and helps to ensure that corrected rotations are maintained. For an improved aesthetic result the acrylic used can be a dentine shade.

Begg retainer

This retainer, which was devised for the Begg technique, avoids the need for a molar clasp by using a continuous bow with adjustment loops which emerges distal to the upper molars (Figure 11.3). This appliance has the advantage that the absence of the molar clasps permits better settling of the occlusion but, for the same reason, good appliance retention may be difficult to achieve.

Vacuum-formed retainers

The advent of newer materials has enabled vacuum-formed retainers to be made. These are inconspicuous and excellent at retaining rotations or apical position of incisors. A full arch coverage, however, prevents settling of the buccal occlusion and any closure of slight residual extraction space. A retainer extending only

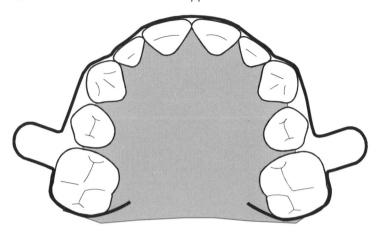

Figure 11.3 A Begg retainer with a continuous labial bow and 'U' loops (0.8 mm).

from canine to canine might permit spontaneous improvements in the buccal segments but would also carry a possible risk of inhalation.

Bonded retainers

Direct acid-etched bonding technique allows groups of teeth to be bonded together on the lingual or palatal side. Commercial retainers are available and are particularly suited to holding two upper central incisors together or maintaining lower anterior tooth position when bonded to the lower canines. These devices are less satisfactory in controlling multiple rotations and they can, on occasion, result in decalcification or even caries if one side becomes unbonded while the other remains firmly attached.

It is probably better to use custom-made bonded retainers with a multi-flex wire adapted to the palatal surfaces of those teeth to be retained. A flexible plastic template can be made on a vacuum-forming machine as an aid in correct location of the wire in an indirect bonding technique. Such bonding should be done under rubber dam to ensure a dry field (much more difficult to achieve on the lingual than the labial surface) and to guard against accidental inhalation. Chemical or light cured agents can be used to bond these retainers. Once this has been achieved an impression should be taken for a removable retainer either of the 'U' loop or vacuum-formed type, as appropriate, as an additional safeguard. Bonded retainers can be left *in situ* for many years but the patient should be seen from time to time and is given careful instruction to return should any part become unbonded or a

tooth show signs of mobility or relapse. There is evidence that these retainers, like bonded bridges, are much less likely to suffer bond failure when only two teeth are bonded.

Periodontal retainers

Non-metallic fibre strips are commercially available for splinting. They are intended to stabilize teeth that have become mobile because of advanced periodontal disease. Such material can be used for orthodontic retention. It is inclined to spread vertically and encroach on the gingival margins in young patients, particularly in lower incisors. For this reason multistrand wires are to be preferred.

Retention regime

Retention can be divided in to short-term retention, standard retention and long-term retention.

Short-term retention

Following removable appliance treatment to correct a reverse overjet, the existing appliance can be used to act as a retainer, any springs or screws being made passive. The appliance can be worn on nights-only basis for 3–6 months.

Standard retention

Standard retention would involve the fitting of a custom-built retainer which would be worn full time for 6 months, followed by a further 6 months of night-time wear, giving a total of 12 months' retention.

When standard retention is required, it is rarely appropriate to use the last removable appliance. An appliance with flexible springs, such as an apron spring or a Roberts' retractor, is unsuitable for conversion to a retainer because the springs cannot readily be made passive and will deform easily. Purpose-made retainers are usually better for standard retention.

Long-term retention

Long-term retention will be required following the correction of rotations, closure of a median diastema and also where there is doubt about the stability of overjet reduction, perhaps due to the upper lip posture or to existing proclination of the lower labial segment. Long-term retention is also required following a combination of complex treatment using both functional and fixed appliances.

Where long-term retention is required for an adolescent patient it may be wise to continue this until growth is complete, but the deciding factor must still be the clinical response rather than the age of the patient.

When the teeth are clinically firm and the patient reports that the retainer does not feel tight, even when first inserted after being left out for a day or two, wear of the retainer can be reduced to three nights a week. Later, if all seems well, then wear can be further reduced to one or two nights a week before finally being left out. Even then it is a good idea to check the fit of the retainer from time to time, to confirm that there has been no tooth movement. A wise orthodontist never tells his patients to throw away the retainer.

Some adult patients may require permanent retention, but such an intention must be made clear to the patient at the outset of treatment.

Treatment methods

Removable appliances

At the end of removable appliance treatment some residual extraction space may be present. During a patient's growth phase the potential for spontaneous space closure is good but a conventional retainer may have the disadvantage of preventing space closure while it maintains the corrected tooth positions. The need to clasp teeth makes it difficult to design a retainer which will permit continuing space closure and by the time retention is complete much potential for closure may have been lost so that space remains. A compromise must be reached between these two conflicting requirements and careful judgement is necessary. In cases where residual space is expected it may be wise to allow some spontaneous closure to occur after the initial extractions before the commencement of active treatment. In cases of doubt a vacuum-formed retainer which only retains the labial segments can be useful to maintain a reduced overjet while leaving the buccal teeth free to move forwards and close the residual spaces.

Functional appliances

Following functional appliance therapy with an Andresen or activator type of appliance the retention follows much the same rules as for single arch removable appliances. Hours of wear can be reduced gradually. It is often necessary to trim the acrylic to allow the buccal teeth to settle into a comfortable class I intercuspation. Any type of functional appliance may produce some proclination of the lower labial segment so the alignment of the lower labial segment must be carefully watched during the retention phase because the teeth may be in an unstable position. It is likely that this tendency to relapse will remain however long retention is maintained.

Fixed appliance treatment

Removable retainers are routinely used in upper and lower arches following fixed appliance treatment. Progressive withdrawal of the appliances following the end of a year of retention is almost invariably undertaken.

Fixed appliances are associated with the treatment of difficult malocclusions or of significant local problems. Two types of tooth movement are especially prone to relapse: rotations and space closure. Rotated teeth need a long period of careful retention after alignment.

During a complex treatment de-rotation will usually be carried out early so that the fixed appliance itself will often retain the corrected rotations for a year or more before a removable retainer is fitted. This may help to reduce any post-treatment relapse. When the correction of rotation is the main tooth movement the treatment time is likely to be shorter and relapse is much more likely.

A number of techniques have been used to stabilize rotations after fixed appliance therapy. A removable 'U' loop retainer is not very effective at maintaining rotations after correction by fixed appliances. Even a fitted labial bow with bends mesial and distal to the rotated tooth is not effective in controlling a rotation and the most satisfactory design is a labial bow with an acrylic cover which engages firmly on the labial surface of the teeth. An alternative is to use a vacuum-formed semi-rigid splint of clear plastic. This is more effective than a conventional labial wire on a retainer because it provides intimate contact with the whole crown of the tooth. The fact that the occlusal surfaces of the teeth are covered represents a disadvantage because it prevents the 'settling in' of the upper and lower posterior teeth when this is required. Each case must be judged on its merits. The priority during the early months must be the maintenance of any corrected rotations. Once confidence in the stability of this aspect is gained a vacuum-formed retainer may be discarded in favour of a 'U' loop retainer. Surgery in the form of pericision can help to stabilize treated rotations, but if it is required for more than one or two teeth it can become a traumatic procedure, especially for a young patient.

Spaces which have been closed pose special problems for retention. The stability of extraction site closure is enhanced when the roots are parallel and the upper and lower posterior teeth have good intercuspation at the end of treatment. The upper mid-line space presents the greatest challenge. Even vacuum-formed retainers will not hold these spaces closed without other forms of retention. Two other techniques are available to aid the retention of rotations and closed spaces – surgery and acid etched bonded retaining wires. In attempting to control upper mid-line spaces (diastemas), fraenectomy has been popular. Fraenectomy before orthodontic treatment has been shown to have little effect but may be useful following space closure with fixed appliances. Gingival surgery can also be useful to improve the appearance by reshaping the gingival contour. Tissue compressed in the mid-line is a potent factor in the re-opening of mid-line spaces and in such cases it is wise to be fairly radical, removing the fraenum, reshaping the gingivae and perhaps sectioning the transeptal fibres. Even after this procedure other forms of retention will be required.

A disadvantage of fixed retainers is that the ultimate responsibility for their care rests with the practitioner and if many patients have such retainers this may become onerous. A removable retainer is more fairly the patient's responsibility, only requiring professional assistance in the event of loss or damage. This does not have the same degree of urgency as a broken or loose bonded retainer.

Retention is important. The more experienced the orthodontist the more cautious he or she is likely to be about retention. Few patients complain about retainer wear (fixed or removable) but almost all are disappointed by relapse, sometimes when only very small tooth movements are involved. At the outset of a course of orthodontic treatment these factors should be explained to the patient who should also be warned that a small degree of relapse must be expected in many cases despite the most careful postoperative care.

References

Little, R.M., Reidel, R.A., Artun, J. (1988) An evaluation of changes in mandibular anterior alignment from 10 to 20 years post-retention. *American Journal of Orthodontics*, **93**: 423–428

Further reading

Otuyemi, P., Jones, S. (1995) Long term evaluation of treated Class II division I malocclusions utilising the PAR index. *British Journal of Orthodontics*, **22**: 171–178

Chapter 12

Problem cases

This chapter deals with a number of situations, many of which will demand fixed appliances if satisfactory results are to be achieved. In certain situations, however, judiciously planned extractions and the use of removable appliances may produce worthwhile improvements.

Missing teeth and teeth with abnormal form

Missing upper laterals

Absence of an upper lateral incisor may be suspected when the deciduous tooth is absent or if its loss is delayed. If the permanent tooth does not erupt, radiographic investigation is required.

Where both upper laterals are congenitally absent and there is a degree of crowding, interceptive extraction of the upper deciduous laterals and deciduous canines may encourage forward eruption of the permanent canines, so allowing them to make contact with the central incisors. Where only one of the lateral incisors is missing, a less satisfactory result is likely to be obtained. The possibility of a centre-line shift may make it preferable to plan treatment involving prosthetic replacement of the missing lateral incisor at a later stage. An older patient with a missing lateral incisor will usually require fixed appliances. In the presence of crowding and distally inclined canines, however, it may occasionally be possible to tilt the canines mesially with a removable appliance – so bringing them into contact with the central incisors.

Peg-shaped upper lateral incisors

These have an unattractive appearance and can be difficult to restore satisfactorily. Attempts to move the posterior teeth forward to close space may result in an unsatisfactory buccal intercuspation. Where there is sufficient crowding, extraction of peg-shaped lateral incisors may be considered, but removable appliances are only suited to deal with this problem when the canines are distally inclined and can be tipped into contact with the centrals.

Missing lower incisors

Lower central incisors are occasionally absent, with the deciduous incisors being retained. In the absence of marked crowding it is usually advisable to retain the deciduous incisors until such time as they can be satisfactorily restored or replaced. Where crowding is present it is sometimes possible to extract the deciduous incisors and later the deciduous canines to encourage forward movement of the lower buccal segments and assist space closure.

Missing second premolars

Second premolars are commonly congenitally absent. This may be detected as part of a general dental examination between the age of 9 and 10 years, so that interceptive extractions can be considered. In a crowded lower arch, early extraction of the deciduous canine and first deciduous molar can be considered to promote forward movement of the second deciduous molar and lower first molar. Where the congenital absence is unilateral, consideration may have to be given to a compensating permanent tooth extraction on the opposite side, possibly of the lower first premolar. In the absence of marked crowding unilateral loss may be acceptable with acceptance of some centre-line shift, although this may mean that it will not be possible to obtain a satisfactory buccal intercuspation. In many cases of congenital absence of the lower second premolars the use of fixed appliances is indicated.

In the upper arch, congenital absence of the upper second premolars may sometimes be managed with removable appliances – the second deciduous molars being retained until such time as space is required. The upper second deciduous molars are then extracted and removable appliances used to retract the first premolars and canines as appropriate. This gives less space than the extraction of upper first premolars and there is less likely to be a satisfactory contact between the first premolar and first molar than there is between a canine and second premolar following conventional first premolar extractions. Where space requirements are large, perhaps due to a combination of crowding and an increased overjet, extraoral forces may be required to maintain the anchorage during the premolar and canine retraction.

Traumatic loss of anterior teeth

The traumatic loss of a central incisor is common and if it is not possible to re-implant the tooth, a removable space maintainer should be fitted immediately. This should carry a prosthetic tooth to maintain the space. Stainless steel spurs on the mesial aspects of the adjacent incisors will also help to prevent these teeth from encroaching on the space (Figure 12.1). Once the space is maintained a decision can be taken concerning the long-term management of the case. Movement of the lateral incisor into the central incisor space prior to preparing a conversion crown on the lateral incisor is unsatisfactory. It is difficult to make a crowned lateral on one side of the arch match a natural central and lateral on the opposite side of the arch.

Occasionally, when both central incisors are missing or traumatized, it may be appropriate to approximate the laterals before crowning them. Such movement is beyond the scope of removable appliances and requires fixed appliance management.

Traumatic loss of lower incisors, unless there is appropriate crowding and distal inclination of the lower canines, is likely to require either fixed appliances or prosthetic restoration.

Where crowding is present, space from a lost lower incisor may well close spontaneously, but will probably give an unsatisfactory buccal

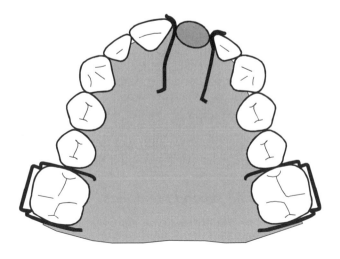

Figure 12.1 An appliance to hold space for a traumatically lost central incisor. Stainless steel spurs are placed on either side of the missing incisor to prevent space loss. Prosthetic replacement for 1|.

segment relationship due to the discrepancy in the number of teeth in each arch.

Non-vital teeth

Non-vital teeth may be moved orthodontically, provided that they have been adequately root filled and have a reasonable root length. The patient and parents should be warned that it is possible for such teeth to become excessively mobile or to resorb during treatment. Gentle forces must be used; a check on tooth mobility should be made regularly and radiographs taken if necessary.

Where a tooth is traumatized but remains vital, orthodontic movement may cause loss of vitality. Following a history of trauma the child's parents should be warned of this possibility before orthodontic treatment commences.

Enforced extractions

The need to extract teeth as the result of caries has reduced greatly in recent years. First molars may still present problems on occasion either due to caries or hypoplasia.

Provided that all unerupted premolars and second molars are present, the early extraction of lower first molars can give good results in a crowded case. Usually, such extractions will demand compensating upper first molar extractions to avoid the over-eruption of the upper first molar, which might interfere with space closure in the lower arch. In the established dentition, extraction of the lower first molars will invariably require the use of a fixed appliance to achieve satisfactory space closure and alignment.

In the upper arch, a limited amount of tooth movement can be achieved following the extraction of upper first molars. This does not give sufficient room to reduce an overjet. In a class I case, movement of the premolars into the first molar extraction site can give space to align canines.

Where the upper first molars must be extracted before the eruption of second molars it may be difficult to provide adequate retention. The problem may be overcome by retaining one of the first molars temporarily to accept a clasp, while the opposite first molar is extracted and the premolars retracted to relieve crowding. Once this is completed a new appliance will be required, clasping the premolars and the second molar, while the opposite first molar is extracted and further tooth movement carried out. This will, inevitably, lengthen treatment.

Where there is marked crowding or a significant overjet to be reduced, it may be more sensible to extract the upper first molars, allow spontaneous space closure and consider further extractions at a later stage.

Centre-line shift

A shift of the centre-line may occur following unilateral early loss of a deciduous tooth, whether this has occurred spontaneously or as the result of enforced extraction. Unilateral loss of a permanent tooth, for example a first molar, may also produce a centre-line shift. This tends to be more noticeable in the upper arch, but is just as significant in the lower arch. Maintenance of a correct centre-line in the lower arch is important if a satisfactory buccal intercuspation is to be achieved at the end of treatment. Balancing extractions should be considered, especially in the lower arch, if there is an element of crowding. In the upper arch, correction of a shifted centre-line cannot be achieved with a removable appliance.

An apparent shift of the lower centre-line may be due to a displacing activity of the mandible associated with a buccal crossbite. The initial treatment will usually involve elimination of the displacing activity by means of upper arch expansion before the extraction of any permanent teeth is considered (see Chapter 7).

Unilateral crowding

Occasionally, marked crowding may be present on one side of the arch. If this is associated with a centre-line shift then unilateral extraction may allow the shift to worsen, especially in a growing child. Unilateral extraction can be considered in an established dentition or in an adult.

Where unilateral crowding is present in the absence of a centre-line shift then premolar extractions may be considered at the site of crowding.

Many such cases, however, are best treated by the extraction of first premolars on the side of the crowding, second premolars on the opposite side and the use of full fixed appliances. Specialist advice may be advisable in any case where unilateral extractions are being considered.

Further reading

Brezniak, N., Wassertein, A. (1993) Root resorption after orthodontic treatment. *American Journal of Orthodontics*, **103**: 138–146

Dacre, J. (1985) The long term effects of one lower incisor extraction. *European Journal of Orthodontics*, **7**: 136–144

Appendix 1

Laboratory procedures

Removable appliances can perform only limited tooth movements. They are simple and it is often assumed that their design and construction demand little thought. This is untrue – and especially so because a removable appliance has limited adaptability. The mode of action of a fixed appliance, for example, may be totally altered by changing the type or form of the archwire, by adding hooks, power-chains and auxiliaries, or by introducing intra- or intermaxillary elastics. A removable appliance, by contrast, is designed to carry out a limited number of specific tasks and is constructed in the laboratory to this end. The need to alter its mode of action will often require a return to the laboratory – involving expense and the need for a further appointment, which is inconvenient to the patient.

It is most important that every appliance is designed to be as effective and trouble free as possible and this implies a good working relationship between the laboratory and the clinician.

Design

The appliance should ideally be designed while the patient is still in the chair. This allows teeth to be inspected for their suitability for clasping and permits them to be checked in occlusion and the position of muscle attachments to be located. To design an appliance from the 'mirror-image' presented by an impression carries obvious risks.

It is best to use a standard design-form agreed with the laboratory. (An example of a design form is shown on page 112.) Ideally, this should allow the prescription to be written and the design to be drawn. It is sensible to adopt a routine sequence for design. For example, one might commence by specifying retentive wirework before going on to active springs. Next would come additions such as screws or prosthetic teeth and finally any adaptations or extensions necessary to the baseplate. Wire dimensions should normally be stated unless they are to standards accepted by the clinician and the laboratory. It goes almost without saying that legibility brings benefits to all those involved.

The appliance should be designed to carry out a limited number of tasks and retention should be planned in the light of these tasks. An embrasure will usually afford space to accept a single wire but will rarely accept two wires and appliances are best designed to avoid this.

The impression for a working model should be sufficiently extended to show all teeth that may impinge on the appliance, to reveal the full vault of the palate, to provide good sulcus depth and to demonstrate any muscle attachments. An impression that contains sizeable air-blows, has distorted or has come away from the tray must be retaken. To avoid the risk of cross-infection it is recommended that the impressions should be rinsed briefly under the tap immediately after being removed from the mouth and then disinfected by immersion for

THE ORTHODONTIC LABORATORY

Laboratory Ref.............................. Cast Ref...................

Practice.........................Dental Surgeon.........................Patient.........................Date.........................Box Number................

Please construct removable/fixed orthodontic appliance to the following instructions:

Teeth to be extracted   Date Required..

KEEP AWAY FROM EXTREMES OF HEAT OR COLD

Received by..Constructed by..Released by..

10 minutes in a hypochlorite solution. It should be indicated to the laboratory that this has been carried out.

The laboratory

Ideally, the laboratory should be close at hand to the surgery so that there is regular contact between the two and misunderstandings are minimized. Where this is impossible it is still sensible to try to build a good relationship with the laboratory so that praise can be given and constructive suggestions may be tactfully made. The clinician needs to have confidence in the technician and to know that wirework is constructed with the minimum of bending and that soldered joints have not been annealed.

When impressions must be posted to the laboratory it is important that these are kept damp in sealed polythene bags and that they are well padded and packed to avoid distortion and damage during transit. If an impression for a work model is likely to be subjected to delay it may be more sensible to cast and post the model itself.

The laboratory should return the work model with the appliance so that it may be stored in the patient's model box and will be available in the event of a breakage. Provided that a broken appliance can still be fitted in the mouth it can be replaced on the model to allow clasp replacement or acrylic repair.

Construction

In the past, removable appliances were fully constructed in wax. They were then flasked, boiled out, packed and heat-cured using the same method as for full dentures. Today, they are almost always made using cold-cured acrylic resins, which have been specially formulated for orthodontic use.

The model should initially be inspected and, if necessary, trimmed to allow the arrowheads of the clasps to engage undercuts. The palatal area will then be painted with a mould seal, which is allowed to dry. The wire components – clasps and springs – will be made, positioned on the model and secured in place by flowing wax, melted with a wax-knife, around those parts which will not be embedded in the baseplate. The wax also serves to prevent the acrylic from extending into unwanted areas. For example, where posterior bite planes are to be incorporated into the appliance the acrylic should not enclose the clasp wires where they cross the embrasures.

The acrylic for the baseplate is built up by the alternate application of polymer powder and liquid monomer, generally using a small plastic 'puffer' bottle for the powder and a dropper bottle for the liquid. The resultant mixture has a firm gel-like consistency which does not flow but may be trimmed with a knife. If the model is laid flat there will be a tendency for acrylic to build up in the vault of the palate during construction. This is avoided by resting the model at an angle during construction – turning it around as each section is completed. As with a heat-cured appliance, the palate should be about as thick as a single sheet of baseplate wax. The acrylic can be built up to form anterior or posterior bite planes to the required dimensions.

The completed model is placed in hand-warm water in a pressure flask and left to cure. Subsequently, the appliance may be removed from the model, trimmed, smoothed and polished.

Screws

In the days when appliances were invariably heat-cured, screws had to be 'plastered out'. That is to say that the exposed portion of the screw needed to be covered with plaster so that the wax (and therefore, later, the acrylic) did not flow into this part during construction and obstruct turning. Nowadays, screws are usually supplied with a tag of plastic, which protects the exposed portion. To assist the accurate positioning of the spring a small slot may be cut into the plaster model to seat the screw tag or the screw may be temporarily fixed in place with a dab of sticky wax. Alternatively, some technicians will merely support the screw in place as the acrylic palate is built up. The plastic tag may be removed later. Some screws incorporate a direction marker, which indicates to the patient the direction in which the screw must be turned.

Screws were originally made entirely of metal. Nowadays, some are made with plastic blocks into which the screw thread engages. The elasticity of the plastic allows the screw to engage with slight friction so that the fit is less likely to become floppy as treatment proceeds.

Prosthetic teeth

From time to time it may be necessary to incorporate a prosthetic tooth onto a removable appliance or a retainer. This represents an excellent way of maintaining a space, which will later be restored with a bridge or some other prosthesis. It also makes the appliance more acceptable to the patient. A particular technical problem is that the special cold-cured orthodontic resins are Bis GMA compounds which do not bond well to prosthetic teeth and any tooth is likely to become detached from the appliance. If the tooth is roughened and a small amount of conventional cold-cured acrylic is incorporated between the tooth and the baseplate adhesion will be much improved.

Clasp construction

Accurate wire bending demands practice. It is important that each bend is correct first time. Any substantial correction, which must be made to a bend, work-hardens the wire further and makes it more liable to break later, during use.

Adams' clasps are most commonly constructed from 0.7 mm hard stainless-steel wire, which is ideal for molar clasps. Adams' universal pliers are well suited to this task. Alternatively, a pair of light wire pliers (such as Ormco ABZ 0411 or 6A61) may be used. The stages are as follows:

1. Define the bridge of the clasp by bending the wire to a little beyond a right angle at each end. After the first bend is made the wire can be offered up to the tooth before the second bend is made so that the arrowheads will be correctly situated to grip the tooth and engage undercut at the mesial and distal corners (Figure A.1).
2. The ends of the wire are bent up to form the arrowheads, which are, initially, made in the same plane as the previous bends. Each arrowhead is bent in three stages. The initial bend is made through 90° (Figure A.2). The second bend is best made over the tips of the pliers to permit a sufficiently narrow arrowhead (Figure A.3). The arrowhead must next be pinched up slightly so that its sides are parallel (Figure A.4).
3. The arrowheads must now be bent to an angle of around 45° to the bridge to permit the clasp to sit correctly against the tooth (Figure A.5).
4. The outer arm of the arrowhead should be grasped with the pliers about half way along its length and bent through around 90° so that the free end will rest across the embrasure when the clasp is correctly positioned. This must be done for each side of the clasp. The arrowheads should sit at about 45° to the long axis of the tooth (Figure A.6).
5. Finish off the tags. Each tag will need to be tailored into its embrasure so that it achieves as low a profile as possible and is not traumatized by the opposing teeth. This will usually entail some slight lateral adjustments (Figure A.7). On the palatal side of the contact point the tag should pass down towards the palatal papilla before being kinked slightly away from the plaster. It should then run parallel to the plaster and just out of contact with it for about 1 cm. The end should be cut off and turned down to rest on the model (Figure A.8). This ensures that the wire tag will later be completely surrounded by acrylic during construction. The finished clasp is shown (Figure A.9).

Repairs

Appliance breakage represents an inconvenience to everyone involved and, if repeated, can prolong treatment. Kerr (1984) suggests that most breakages are due to inadequacies of the acrylic or to patient carelessness. In many instances the appliance must be returned to the laboratory for repair, but minor repairs and adjustments can, on occasion, be carried out at the chairside.

Acrylic repair and modifications

Minor fractures to the edges of the acrylic baseplate may be inconsequential. All that is necessary is to smooth the sharp edge with a suitable polishing stone so that it is comfortable to the tongue.

More major acrylic fractures will require the appliance to be re-seated onto the work-model (after this has been treated with a mould seal) before repair. The area adjacent to the break should be cut back and roughened so that additional acrylic may be added before curing and finishing. Such a repair is usually best returned to the laboratory. It may, however, be sensible to reassemble the appliance first, using a cyanoacrylate glue, so that the fit may be checked in the mouth. This will avoid the time and expense involved in arranging a repair, only to discover that the appliance does not fit because it has been out of the mouth for some time before or after the breakage.

When an appliance incorporates a screw which has been turned it will no longer fit the model. In this event the screw will need to be turned back to zero (and the number of turns recorded) before the appliance can be fitted to the model. After repair, the screw may be re-opened before the appliance is refitted in the mouth.

It may often be necessary to build up an anterior bite plane during the course of treatment so that further bite opening can be obtained. This is easily carried out at the chairside using one of the acrylics intended for denture relining or extension. The surface of the existing bite plane is roughened and the acrylic is mixed to a wet dough. It is applied evenly to the bite plane and the appliance is then held in tepid water for a few moments until the acrylic surface has 'skinned'. The

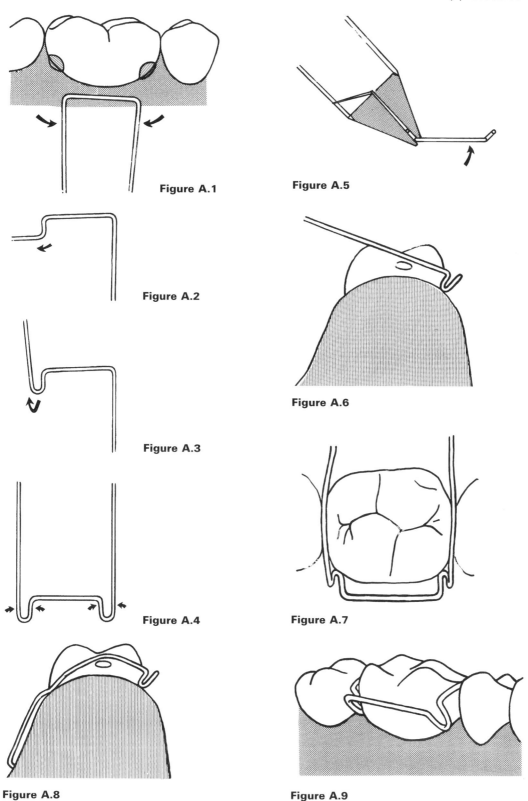

Figure A.1

Figure A.2

Figure A.3

Figure A.4

Figure A.5

Figure A.6

Figure A.7

Figure A.8

Figure A.9

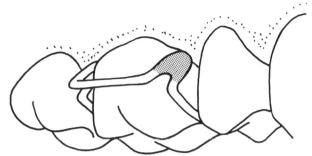

Figure A.10

appliance may then be tried in the mouth and the added acrylic gently shaped with the fingers to the correct level, so that the lower incisors have an even contact. The rest of the curing may be completed in warm water.

Wire fractures

It is occasionally possible to carry out a soldered repair to an Adams' clasp if a fracture has occurred at the tip of the arrowhead, although this is an unusual place for a break unless the wire has been overworked during construction. The arrowhead should be cleaned, fluxed and flushed with solder (Figure A.10). Other attempts to repair a broken clasp are rarely worthwhile and replacement is usually the more sensible option.

On occasion, a clasp that has broken where the wire crosses the embrasure may be cut away to leave one intact arrowhead, which can be pinched closed with a pair of pliers so that no sharp end remains. The arrowhead may be adjusted to provide some retention. This procedure is useful where the retention provided by other wires is fairly good and especially when the appliance is not going to be worn for much longer.

Broken springs may be fairly easily dealt with. The remains of the spring are cut away and a recess drilled into the fitting surface of the acrylic baseplate. A replacement spring may be bent up and embedded into this space using a small amount of cold-cured acrylic. In the case of a palatal finger spring the presence of a guard wire will help to hold the new spring in place during this procedure.

References

Kerr, W.J.S. (1984) Appliance breakages. *British Journal of Orthodontics*, **11**: 137–142

Further reading

Munns, D. (1971) An analysis of broken removable appliances. *Proceedings BSSO*, 45–48

Appendix 2

Instructions for wearing your removable appliance

About your brace

Your removable appliance (brace) consists of an acrylic plate, which covers the roof of your mouth, incorporating wires and springs, to move the teeth.

Initial difficulties

The orthodontist will show you how to put the appliance in and take it out. Practise this before you leave the surgery. At first it will feel very big. You may make extra saliva, find it difficult to swallow and talk. Provided you persevere, these problems will soon improve.

Hours of wear

You must wear your brace **all the time** – except for the following reasons:

Cleaning

Your appliance should be removed after meals for cleaning. It can be cleaned using your toothbrush and toothpaste after you have cleaned your teeth. Alternatively you can use a nail brush with warm soapy water. Pay particular attention to the fitting surface. If you are out and do not have a toothbrush available wash the brace under a cold water tap and rinse your mouth out.

Special cleaners like 'Retainer-brite' are available and effective at cleaning deposits that are difficult to remove with a toothbrush.
Do not put the brace into very hot water or bleach.

Contact-sports and wind instrument playing

If the retainer has to be removed for such activities it must be put into a small rigid plastic container. If you put it in your pocket the springs can easily be damaged or bent.

Replace it in your mouth as soon as you have finished sport or music practice. Braces are often broken or lost while they are out of the mouth.

End of treatment

Once your teeth are in the correct position it may not be necessary to wear the brace full time. Wait until your orthodontist tells you that you have reached this stage.

Eating

The appliance must be worn for meals. This will be difficult initially but you will quickly adapt to it. Please do not chew gum or eat sticky things (like toffee) because these can damage the appliance.

Problems

If your brace is damaged, doesn't fit, hurts or keeps falling out, please contact the orthodontist promptly.

Replacement

If your brace has to be replaced because of carelessness a charge may be made.

Remember! When the appliance is not in your mouth your teeth are not improving. Previous progress can be lost. If you do not wear the brace as instructed we may have to stop your treatment.

Appendix 3

Recommended wire diameters

Retention

Posterior

Adams' clasps 6|6	0.7 mm
Adams' clasps 4|4	0.6 mm
Clasp to engage molar tubes 6|6	0.7 mm
Adams' clasps c|c and d|d	0.6 mm

Anterior

Double Adams' clasp 1|1	0.7 mm
Southend clasp	0.7 mm
Fitted labial bow 21|12	0.7 mm
'c' clasp	0.6 mm

Active components

Buccal

Low labial bow	0.7 mm
Reverse loop labial bow	0.7 mm
Extended labial bow	0.7 mm

Roberts' retractor	0.5 mm in 0.5 mm ID tubing
Apron spring	0.5 mm wound on high labial bow of 0.9 mm
Self-straightening wires	0.5 mm on labial bow 0.7 mm
Buccal canine retractor	a) Self supporting 0.7 mm b) Supported 0.5 mm in 0.5 mm ID tubing
Self-supporting buccal spring to move canines and premolars palatally	0.7 mm

Palatal

Cantilever spring to retract canines and premolars	0.5 mm
Double cantilever ('Z') spring	0.5 mm
'T' spring	0.5 mm
Coffin spring	1.25 mm

Index

Main references are in **bold** type

CD ROM
produced in association
with

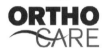

Orthodontic Product Specialists